# ACID REFLUX DIET

# COOKBOOK

# FOR BEGINNERS

Budget-Friendly Recipes and Easy 28 day Meal Plan for relief from Heartburn, GERD, LPR Symptoms and a Healthy Digestive System

## Dorothy S. Richard

# CONTENTS

# INTRODUCTION

Have you ever experienced the scorching feeling of stomach acid moving up your throat, leaving you gasping for breath and dreading your next meal?

If so, you're not alone. Acid reflux, commonly known as gastroesophageal reflux disease (GERD), affects millions of people worldwide, turning even the simplest pleasures of eating into a cause of suffering. But worry not, fellow heartburn sufferers! There's light at the end of the oesophagus, and it's in the shape of this tasty and educational cookbook.

In this Comprehensive book, you'll discover a world of exquisite dishes that not only cure your digestive issues but also excite your taste buds.

Forget bland, monotonous meals; this cookbook is filled with rich tastes and culinary inventiveness, illustrating that acid reflux doesn't have to mean compromising taste. Whether you're seeking a robust breakfast, a delicious lunch, or a tasty supper, you'll find a recipe to fit your mood and palette.

However, this cookbook isn't just about recipes; it's about enabling you to take control of your acid reflux and restore your pleasure of eating. You'll learn about the science behind acid reflux, identify trigger foods, and uncover easy lifestyle modifications that can make a world of difference. With this information, you'll be able to make informed decisions about what you eat and how you live, successfully controlling your symptoms and lowering your need for medication.

So, if you're ready to wave goodbye to heartburn and embrace a life filled with gastronomic pleasures, then continue to read  the remaining pages of "Acid Reflux Diet Cookbook for Beginners" and begin on a road towards heartburn-free joy.

**I guarantee You won't Regret It!**

# PART 1

# UNDERSTANDING ACID REFLUX

# CHAPTER 1: INTRODUCTION TO ACID REFLUX

Gastroesophageal reflux disease (GERD), generally known as acid reflux, is a disorder defined by the backward movement of stomach contents into the oesophagus, leading to symptoms such as heartburn and regurgitation. This happens when the lower oesophageal sphincter, a ring of muscle between the oesophagus and the stomach, fails not shut correctly, enabling stomach acid to leak into the oesophagus

Normally, the oesophagus clears acidic stomach contents by repeated peristalsis and neutralizes them with salivary bicarbonate. However, reduced oesophageal peristalsis can lead to poor clearance of gastric reflux, resulting in severe reflux symptoms and mucosal injury.

GERD is a widespread illness, especially in developed nations, and its prevalence is growing. It can manifest as non-erosive reflux disease or erosive esophagitis, with variable degrees of severity.

High-fat diets, particularly those incorporating fried or greasy meals, are theorized to increase GERD symptoms. Certain foods, such as chocolate, wine, and high-fat meals, might diminish esophageal sphincter pressure and increase esophageal exposure to stomach fluids, worsening GERD symptoms

Treatment for GERD involves lifestyle adjustments, such as dietary changes, weight control, and raising the head of the bed, as well as drugs such as proton pump inhibitors and H2 receptor antagonists.

Knowing the pathophysiology of GERD and its influence on the esophagus is critical in controlling the illness. Additionally, identifying the function of nutrition in worsening or easing symptoms is vital for persons with GERD.

# CHAPTER 2: THE IMPACT OF DIET ON ACID REFLUX

Diet has a crucial impact in managing acid reflux symptoms and is the primary line of treatment utilized for persons with GERD. Certain foods can induce acid reflux symptoms, while others can help avoid them.

Foods that are heavy in fat, salt, or spice, such as fried food, chocolate, peppermint, and carbonated drinks, are known to be heartburn triggers and should be avoided. High-fiber meals, such as whole grains, root vegetables, and green vegetables, can help reduce acid reflux by making you feel full, so you're less inclined to overeat. Alkaline foods, such as bananas, melons, cauliflower, fennel, and almonds, can help balance strong stomach acid.

A comprehensive analysis indicated that ingestion of alcohol, chocolate, and high-fat meals lowers esophageal sphincter pressure and increases esophageal exposure to stomach fluids, which might aggravate GERD symptoms. Therefore, it is advisable to avoid alcohol and high-fat meals.

It is also vital to pay attention when you eat. Digestion increases the quantity of gastric acid present in the stomach, hence it is better to avoid eating right before bed.

A good diet can help avoid acid reflux symptoms. Avoiding heartburn triggers such as high-fat, salt, or spice meals, and alcohol, and including high-fiber and alkaline diets will help reduce acid reflux. It is also crucial to pay attention to when you eat and avoid eating just before bed.

# CHAPTER 3: COMMON SYMPTOMS AND TRIGGERS

Acid reflux, a widespread digestive condition, occurs when stomach acid rushes back into the oesophagus. Understanding its typical signs and triggers is key for successful therapy. Imagine this: you've just indulged in a spicy feast, and suddenly, a scorching feeling creeps up your chest. That's a typical sign of acid reflux - heartburn. However, acid reflux symptoms extend beyond heartburn.

## Common Symptoms

**1. Heartburn**: A burning ache beneath the breastbone is the defining sign. It generally intensifies after meals or while laying down, giving it a clear indicator of acid reflux.

**2. Regurgitation**: Imagine feeling stomach acid in your mouth - that's regurgitation. It's the involuntary return of stomach contents to the throat and happens regularly with acid reflux.

**3. Chest Pain**: Acid reflux might mimic heart pain, producing chest discomfort. This symptom should always be handled carefully, since it may be mistaken with a heart attack.

**4. Dysphagia**: Difficulty swallowing, or dysphagia, can develop from acid-induced inflammation in the oesophagus. It may feel like food is trapped in the throat.

**5. Chronic Cough**: Acid reflux can create a chronic cough, typically misinterpreted for allergies or respiratory disorders. The refluxed stomach acid irritates the airways, resulting in coughing.

Now, let's review the triggers that set the scene for acid reflux episodes:

## Common Triggers

**1. Dietary Culprits**: Spicy and acidic meals, such as tomatoes and citrus fruits, can relax the lower esophageal sphincter (LES), enabling stomach acid to seep into the oesophagus.

**2. Overeating**: A bloated stomach increases pressure on the LES, causing acid reflux. Eating heavy meals or eating close to sleep exacerbates this danger.

**3. Obesity**: Excess weight, particularly around the belly, increases abdominal pressure. This pressure may drive stomach contents into the oesophagus, creating acid reflux.

**4. Hiatal Hernia**: This condition develops when a part of the stomach protrudes through the diaphragm, weakening the LES and promoting acid reflux.

**5. Smoking and Alcohol**: Tobacco smoke irritates the LES, whereas alcohol relaxes it. Both practices lead to an increased risk of acid reflux.

Understanding these symptoms and triggers helps people to make informed lifestyle choices.

The route to treating acid reflux needs a personalized strategy, generally including dietary modifications, weight management, and medication. Stay proactive, stay alert of triggers, and relish a life with fewer flaming interruptions.

# HIATAL HERNIA AND ACID REFLUX

A hiatal hernia is a condition that arises when a portion of the stomach protrudes through a hole in the diaphragm, the muscle that divides the chest from the abdomen. This opening is called the hiatus. In most situations, hiatal hernias do not produce any symptoms. However, in rare situations, they can lead to acid reflux, a condition that develops when stomach acid backs up into the oesophagus, producing heartburn and other symptoms.

A hiatal hernia can induce acid reflux by weakening the lower esophageal sphincter (LES), the valve that stops stomach acid from pouring back into the oesophagus. The LES is positioned at the intersection of the oesophagus and the stomach. When the LES is compromised, it cannot seal correctly, enabling stomach acid to back up into the oesophagus.

## Symptoms of a Hiatal Hernia

Most persons with hiatal hernias do not exhibit any symptoms. However, some individuals may develop symptoms of acid reflux, such as heartburn, sour taste in the mouth, trouble swallowing, and regurgitation. Other symptoms of a hiatal hernia may include:

- Chest pain
- Bloating
- Feeling of fullness after eating Risk Factors for Hiatal Hernia

Anyone can develop a hiatal hernia, however some conditions can increase your risk, including:

- **Age**: Hiatal hernias are more frequent in adults over the age of 50.

- **Obesity**: Excess weight exerts extra strain on the abdomen, which may damage the diaphragm.

- **Pregnancy**: Pregnancy may increase strain on the abdomen, which can potentially weaken the diaphragm.

- **Smoking**: Smoking may harm the LES, making it more prone to malfunction.

- **Heavy lifting**: Heavy lifting may also exert extra strain on the abdomen, which can damage the diaphragm.

# Diagnosis of a Hiatal Hernia

A hiatal hernia can be diagnosed using a number of tests, including:

- **Barium swallow**: This test includes consuming a beverage containing barium, which covers the digestive tract and makes it visible on an X-ray.
- **Upper endoscopy**: This test includes inserting a thin, flexible tube with a camera into the esophagus and stomach to search for abnormalities.
- **Esophageal manometry**: This test measures the pressure in the esophagus to determine the strength of the LES.

## Treatment for Hiatal Hernia and Acid Reflux

Treatment for a hiatal hernia and acid reflux depends on the severity of your symptoms. For mild instances, lifestyle adjustments and over-the-counter drugs may be all that is required. Lifestyle adjustments that may help control acid reflux include:

- Eating smaller, more frequent meals
- Avoiding rich, spicy, and acidic meals
- Losing weight if you are overweight or obese
- Quitting smoking
- Elevating the head of your bed at night
- Over-the-counter drugs that may help reduce heartburn include antacids, H2 blockers, and proton pump inhibitors (PPIs).

For more severe episodes of acid reflux, prescription drugs or surgery can be indicated. Surgery is normally only undertaken if lifestyle modifications and drugs have not been beneficial. The form of surgery most usually used to correct a hiatal hernia is termed **fundoplication**. This operation includes wrapping the upper section of the stomach over the lower segment of the oesophagus to strengthen the LES.

## Prevention of Hiatal Hernia

There is no proven method to avoid a hiatal hernia. However, there are certain things you can do to lower your risk, such as:

- Maintaining a healthy weight
- Avoiding heavy lifting
- Quitting smoking

## Living with a Hiatal Hernia

Most persons with hiatal hernias can live regular, healthy lives. With correct therapy, you can control your symptoms and avoid consequences.

Hiatal hernia is a frequent ailment that can cause acid reflux. If you are having symptoms of acid reflux, it is crucial to consult your doctor to acquire a diagnosis and treatment plan. With correct therapy, you can control your symptoms and avoid consequences.

# VAGUS NERVE IMBALANCE AND ACID REFLUX

The vagus nerve is the longest and most complicated nerve in the body. It is part of the parasympathetic nerve system, which is responsible for "rest and digest" tasks. The vagus nerve goes from the brain stem down to the belly, innervating various organs along the route, including the oesophagus, stomach, and intestines.

Vagus nerve imbalance is a condition in which the vagus nerve is not working normally. This can be caused by a variety of circumstances, including stress, anxiety, trauma, and some drugs. Vagus nerve imbalance can contribute to a multitude of symptoms, including acid reflux, heartburn, bloating, and constipation.

## How Does Vagus Nerve Imbalance Cause Acid Reflux?

The vagus nerve serves a crucial function in controlling digestion. It helps to manage the passage of food through the digestive tract and the release of stomach acid. When the vagus nerve is not working correctly, it can lead to poor digestion and an increased risk of acid reflux. There are a few distinct ways in which vagus nerve imbalance might lead to acid reflux:

**Reduced Esophageal Motility**: The vagus nerve serves to govern the muscles in the oesophagus that transport food down into the stomach. When the vagus nerve is not working correctly, these muscles may become weak and slow, which can cause stomach acid to back up into the oesophagus.

**Increased Stomach Acid Production**: The vagus nerve also serves to regulate the secretion of stomach acid. When the vagus nerve is not working correctly, it can lead to an increase in stomach acid production, which can also contribute to acid reflux.

**Relaxed Lower Esophageal Sphincter (LES):** The LES is a muscular valve that divides the oesophagus from the stomach. It helps to prevent stomach acid from backing up into the oesophagus. When the vagus nerve is not working correctly, it can cause the LES to become relaxed, which can also raise the risk of acid reflux.

## Symptoms of Vagus Nerve Imbalance

In addition to acid reflux, vagus nerve imbalance can also induce a variety of other symptoms, including:

- Bloating Constipation
- Diarrhea
- Difficulty swallowing
- Heartburn
- Nausea
- Vomiting
- Fatigue
- Anxiety
- Depression
- Difficulty sleeping

## Risk Factors for Vagus Nerve Imbalance

Anyone can have vagus nerve imbalance, although some circumstances can raise your risk, including:

- Stress
- Anxiety
- Trauma
- Certain drugs
- Autoimmune disorders
- Inflammatory conditions
- Chronic pain

## Diagnosis of Vagus Nerve Imbalance

There is no one test that can detect vagus nerve imbalance. However, your doctor may perform a variety of tests to rule out other probable diseases and examine the function of your vagus nerve. These tests may include:

- Heart rate variability (HRV) test
- Baroreceptor sensitivity test
- Tilt table test
- Gastric emptying study Upper endoscopy

## Treatment for Vagus Nerve Imbalance

Treatment for vagus nerve imbalance relies on the underlying cause and the severity of your symptoms. Treatment options can include:

**Lifestyle Changes**: This includes controlling stress, getting adequate sleep, eating a balanced diet, and exercising frequently.

**Therapy**: This may enable you to manage stress and anxiety, which can help to increase vagus nerve function.

**Medication**: There are a variety of drugs that may be used to treat the symptoms of vagus nerve imbalance, such as antidepressants, anxiolytics, and prokinetics.

**Vagus nerve stimulation (VNS)**: This is a sort of treatment that employs electrical impulses to stimulate the vagus nerve. VNS has been demonstrated to be beneficial in treating a range of disorders, including vagus nerve imbalance.

## Prevention of Vagus Nerve Imbalance

There is no guaranteed method to avoid vagus nerve imbalance, however there are several things you can do to lower your risk, such as:

- Managing stress
- Getting enough sleep
- Eating a healthy diet
- Exercising regularly
- Maintaining a healthy weight

## Living with Vagus Nerve Imbalance

Most persons with vagus nerve imbalance can live regular, healthy lives. With correct therapy, you can control your symptoms and avoid consequences.

# CHAPTER 4: PH IMPACT OF FOODS ON ACID REFLUX

The pH influence of meals on acid reflux is a complicated but crucial factor to know for individuals seeking successful treatment of this digestive pain. Let's dig into the subtleties of pH, the acidity scale, and how our food choices might impact acid reflux.

**Understanding pH:**

pH quantifies the acidity or alkalinity of a material on a scale from 0 to 14. Lower numbers imply acidity, whereas higher values represent alkalinity. The stomach is inherently acidic, with a pH range from 1.5 to 3.5, mostly owing to the hydrochloric acid it generates during digestion. This acidic environment is vital for breaking down food and eliminating dangerous germs.

**Impact of pH on Acid Reflux**:

The lower esophageal sphincter (LES) is a muscular ring dividing the stomach and the oesophagus. Its job is to prevent stomach contents, particularly acid, from going back into the oesophagus. However, some circumstances, particularly the pH of ingested meals, might impact the integrity of the LES.

**Low pH Foods (Acidic):**

Foods with low pH values, such as citrus fruits (lemons, oranges), tomatoes, and vinegar, are innately acidic. Consuming them may lead to a more acidic stomach environment. While acidic meals don't directly damage the LES, they may irritate the esophageal lining, making it more sensitive to the corrosive effects of stomach acid. Individuals prone to acid reflux should reduce their consumption of these acidic meals, particularly in the evening or close to sleep when reflux risk is highest.

**High pH Foods (Alkaline):**

Conversely, foods with higher pH values, generally termed alkaline, include some vegetables (leafy greens, broccoli) and fruits (bananas, melons). These foods may have a neutralizing impact on stomach acid. While they won't suddenly cure acid reflux, integrating alkaline foods into the diet may help balance the overall pH and give relief for some people.

**Water's Neutral pH:**

Pure water has a neutral pH of 7.0. It neither adds to acidity or alkalinity in the stomach. Drinking water between meals or while having heartburn might help dilute stomach acid and alleviate pain. However, excessive water drinking during meals may dilute stomach acid excessively, thereby inhibiting optimal digestion.

**Meal Composition Matters**:

The mix of items in a meal may determine its overall pH effect. For example, a lunch high in acidic foods may have a more dramatic influence on stomach acidity than a balanced meal combining alkaline and neutral meals. Striking a balance and being conscious of individual tolerances is crucial.

**Individual Variability**:

It's crucial to know that people may respond differently to certain meals. While some meals are commonly linked with acidity or alkalinity, personal tolerance levels might differ. Keeping a food journal to document symptoms with dietary choices might help uncover particular causes for acid reflux in a customized way.

The pH effect of meals on acid reflux is a dynamic interaction impacted by the intrinsic acidity of foods, meal composition, and individual variability. A tailored, holistic strategy addressing the pH factor, along with other lifestyle adjustments, may assist greatly in treating acid reflux effectively.

# CHAPTER 5. DISTINGUISHING BETWEEN LPR AND GERD

Distinguishing between LPR (Laryngopharyngeal Reflux) and GERD (Gastroesophageal Reflux Disease) is critical for correct diagnosis and efficient therapy of these related but separate disorders. While both entail the regurgitation of stomach contents into the upper digestive system, they present with distinct symptoms and may damage separate sections of the body.

# Understanding GERD

GERD is a chronic illness defined by the backward passage of stomach acid into the oesophagus. The lower esophageal sphincter (LES), a muscular ring at the intersection of the oesophagus and stomach, generally prevents this reflux. However, when the LES is compromised or relaxes incorrectly, stomach acid may irritate the ocsophagus, leading to symptoms including heartburn, regurgitation, chest discomfort, and trouble swallowing.

## Key GERD Symptoms:

**1. Heartburn**: A burning feeling behind the breastbone is a classic symptom of GERD. It commonly happens after meals or after resting down.

**2. Regurgitation**: Backflow of stomach contents into the oesophagus, occasionally reaching the mouth, may give an unpleasant taste.

**3. Chest Discomfort**: GERD-related chest discomfort may mirror heart-related pain, prompting thorough examination.

4. Dysphagia: Difficulty swallowing may occur from esophageal inflammation.

## Understanding LPR

LPR, on the other hand, includes the reflux of stomach contents into the larynx (voice box) and pharynx (throat). Unlike GERD, LPR generally lacks the characteristic heartburn symptom, making it hard to diagnose. The stomach acid's interaction with the sensitive tissues of the neck and voice box might lead to a particular set of symptoms.

## Key LPR Symptoms:

**1. Hoarseness**: Persistent hoarseness or changes in voice quality are frequent LPR signs.

**2. Chronic Cough**: LPR may generate a chronic cough, typically misdiagnosed as allergies or respiratory disorders.

**3. Throat Clearing**: Frequent throat clearing is a reaction to discomfort induced by stomach acid.

**4. Globus Sensation**: A sense of a lump or foreign object in the neck may be experienced.

**5. Postnasal Drip**: Stomach acid reaching the upper airways might lead to postnasal drip and throat discomfort.

## Differentiating Factors

**1. Symptom Profile**: While heartburn is a significant symptom in GERD, LPR tends to present with throat-related symptoms including hoarseness and recurrent cough.

**2. Diagnostic Challenges**: Diagnosing LPR might be problematic owing to the lack of conventional GERD symptoms. Specialized diagnostics like pH monitoring and laryngoscopy may be required.

**3. Treatment Approaches**: While lifestyle adjustments and drugs like proton pump inhibitors (PPIs) are routinely utilized for both illnesses, the focus on particular therapies may vary. LPR treatment frequently requires behavioral and nutritional modifications, along with avoiding late-night meals.

**4. Impact on the Upper Respiratory Tract**:
LPR's principal effect is on the throat and voice
box, while GERD largely affects the oesophagus.

Differentiating between LPR and GERD
includes identifying the various symptom
profiles and comprehending the sections of the
upper digestive tract impacted. This detailed
knowledge is critical for accurate diagnosis and
developing successful treatment approaches,
underlining the necessity for a holistic strategy
to address the intricacies of various reflux-
related disorders.

# CHAPTER 6. DIAGNOSIS AND RECOMMENDED MEDICAL TESTS

Diagnosing acid reflux needs a systematic method that incorporates patient history, symptom assessment, and, where appropriate, specialized medical testing. Given the diverse manifestations of acid reflux, a detailed diagnosis provides focused and successful care. Here's an in-depth explanation of the diagnosis procedure and a list of suggested medical tests:

## Patient History and Symptom Evaluation

The diagnostic process frequently starts with a detailed patient history. Healthcare practitioners ask about symptoms, their frequency, duration, and any triggering or relieving circumstances. Common acid reflux symptoms including heartburn, regurgitation, chest discomfort, and trouble swallowing are rigorously analyzed. It's vital for people to offer specific information on their lifestyle, food habits, and any circumstances that may increase or relieve symptoms.

## List of Recommended Medical Tests for Acid Reflux

**1. Upper Endoscopy (EGD)**

**Purpose**: To visually evaluate the oesophagus, stomach, and the upper section of the small intestine.

**Procedure**: A thin, flexible tube containing a light and camera (endoscope) is introduced via the mouth into the oesophagus. It permits the healthcare professional to check the lining of the digestive system for symptoms of inflammation, irritation, or injury.

## 2. Esophageal pH Monitoring

**Purpose**: Measures the acidity level in the oesophagus over a time to measure the frequency and duration of acid exposure.

**Procedure**: A tiny tube is placed via the nose or mouth into the oesophagus, and a pH monitor is connected. The patient maintains a journal of symptoms while the equipment collects pH levels.

## 3. Esophageal Manometry

**Purpose**: Evaluates the function of the lower esophageal sphincter (LES) and the muscular contractions of the oesophagus.

**Procedure**: A tiny tube is inserted via the nose into the oesophagus. The tube incorporates pressure sensors to detect muscle contractions while the patient swallows.

## 4. Barium Swallow Test (Esophagram)

**Purpose**: Visualizes the oesophagus and stomach using X-rays after consuming a contrast substance (barium).

**Procedure**: The patient consumes a barium solution, and X-rays are performed to discover anomalies such as strictures or hiatal hernias.

## 5. Ambulatory pH Monitoring

**Purpose**: Similar to esophageal pH monitoring but conducted over a much prolonged time, generally 24 hours.

**Procedure**: A tiny pH monitor is implanted in the oesophagus and linked to a recorder worn by the patient. This gives a more thorough assessment of acid exposure throughout everyday activities.

## 6. Impedance Testing

**Purpose**: Measures the passage of gas and liquids throughout the oesophagus, helping diagnose reflux episodes without relying entirely on pH values.

**Procedure**: Similar to pH monitoring, impedance testing includes the insertion of a tube into the oesophagus.

## 7. Gastric Emptying Study

**Purpose**: Assesses how rapidly the stomach empties its contents into the small intestine.

**Procedure**: The patient takes a meal containing a tiny quantity of radioactive material, and a scanner records the transit of the substance through the digestive system.

## Diagnostic Significance

These tests are crucial for diagnosing acid reflux, assessing its severity, and detecting any consequences. Upper endoscopy offers direct vision of damage, while pH monitoring and impedance tests give objective data on acid exposure. Esophageal manometry examines the functioning of the LES and esophageal contractions, revealing insights into motility disorders.

The diagnostic method for acid reflux involves a combination of patient history, symptom assessment, and specialized diagnostics. This multidimensional approach guarantees a full knowledge of the disease, permitting individualized and successful treatment regimens for those suffering acid reflux symptoms.

# CHAPTER 7: ULTIMATE SUPPLEMENTS AND NATURAL REMEDIES

Supplements can be beneficial complements to lifestyle adjustments and medication therapies for treating acid reflux. While it's vital to contact with a healthcare practitioner before introducing supplements, here's a fresh and extensive analysis of some of the greatest supplements for acid reflux:

**1. Melatonin:** Melatonin, largely recognized for regulating sleep, also demonstrates gastroprotective benefits by lowering stomach acid output and aiding the repair of the esophageal lining. Taking melatonin supplements can lead to increased sleep quality and may be decrease acid reflux symptoms.

**2. Deglycyrrhizinated Licorice (DGL):** DGL, a type of licorice with glycyrrhizin removed, helps increase the creation of mucus in the oesophagus, providing a protective coating against stomach acid. Chewing DGL pills before meals may calm the oesophagus and reduce discomfort.

**3. Probiotics**: Probiotics support a healthy balance of gut bacteria, modulating digestion and perhaps lowering the risk of acid reflux by maintaining a stable gut environment. Consuming probiotic-rich foods like yogurt or taking probiotic supplements can significantly improve gut health.

**4. Ginger**: Ginger contains anti-inflammatory characteristics that can help decrease inflammation in the oesophagus and limit the formation of stomach acid. Drinking ginger tea or taking ginger pills can help relief from acid reflux symptoms.

**5. Magnesium**: Magnesium helps the lower esophageal sphincter (LES) operate appropriately, limiting the reflux of stomach acid into the esophagus. Taking magnesium supplements under the advice of a healthcare practitioner can contribute to LES health.

**6. L-Glutamine**: L-Glutamine is an amino acid that stimulates the regeneration of the mucous lining of the oesophagus, protecting it from acid damage. Including L-Glutamine supplements in the diet can assist in esophageal tissue healing.

It's vital to remember that although certain supplements show potential, individual reactions differ. Consulting with a healthcare practitioner is vital to establish the most suitable vitamins and doses depending on individual health problems and possible interactions with other drugs.

Supplements should complement, not replace, a complete strategy that includes dietary alterations, lifestyle changes, and any recommended drugs for efficient acid reflux treatment.

# NATURAL REMEDIES

Natural therapies can provide helpful alternatives or complements to established treatments for acid reflux. These cures frequently concentrate on lifestyle modifications, dietary improvements, and holistic techniques. Here's a full analysis of several unique and efficient natural therapies for acid reflux:

1. **Aloe Vera:** Aloe vera contains anti-inflammatory qualities that help soothe and decrease discomfort in the oesophagus. It may also assist with digestion and improve healing. Consuming aloe vera juice, prepared for internal use, in moderation can help decrease acid reflux symptoms.

**2. Slippery Elm**: Slippery elm creates a soothing gel when combined with water, providing a protective covering for the oesophagus and stomach lining. Drinking slippery elm tea or taking supplements could help relieve the pain associated with acid reflux.

**3. Chamomile:** Chamomile contains anti-inflammatory and antioxidant characteristics, which may help decrease esophageal irritation and acidity. Sipping on chamomile tea before sleep may encourage calm and maybe relieve overnight acid reflux problems.

**4. Dietary Fiber**: Foods high in fiber, such as whole grains, fruits, and vegetables, encourage regular bowel movements and reduce excessive pressure on the stomach, lowering the probability of acid reflux. Including more fiber-rich foods in the diet, including oatmeal and brown rice, may help to digestive health.

**5. Baking Soda**: Baking soda, or sodium bicarbonate, may serve as a natural antacid, neutralizing stomach acid. Mixing a tiny quantity of baking soda with water and drinking it sometimes may offer brief relief from acid reflux symptoms. However, it's recommended to utilize this medication carefully owing to its high salt concentration.

**6. Gum Chewing**: Chewing gum promotes saliva production, which helps neutralize stomach acid and clear it from the oesophagus. Opting for sugar-free gum after meals may enhance saliva flow and assist in acid reflux avoidance.

**7. Lifestyle Modifications**: Making lifestyle modifications such as maintaining a healthy weight, avoiding tight clothes, and raising the head of the bed may relieve pressure on the stomach and limit the risk of acid reflux. Wearing loose-fitting garments and utilizing bed risers to raise the head of the bed by 6 to 8 inches may help to improve acid reflux control.

**8. Ginger and Turmeric**: Both ginger and turmeric have anti-inflammatory characteristics that may help calm the oesophagus and lessen acid reflux symptoms. Incorporating ginger and turmeric into meals or ingesting them as teas may give natural comfort.

It's vital to seek natural therapies with caution and under the advice of a healthcare practitioner. While many therapies show promise, individual reactions might vary, and over reliance on specific cures may have detrimental consequences. Combining natural treatments with a well-balanced diet, frequent exercise, and keeping a healthy lifestyle gives a comprehensive strategy for controlling acid reflux symptoms successfully. Always speak with a healthcare expert to verify the selected natural therapies correspond with specific health circumstances and requirements.

# PART 2

---

# FOUNDATIONS OF A REFLUX-FRIENDLY DIET

# CHAPTER 8: PRINCIPLES OF AN ACID REFLUX DIET

Crafting a good acid reflux diet entails knowing the principles that govern food choices to reduce symptoms and enhance digestive health. This strategy focuses on regulating the components that lead to acid reflux, such as the lower esophageal sphincter (LES) function, stomach acidity, and overall digestion processes. Here are innovative and thorough concepts for an acid reflux diet:

**1. Low-Acid Foods**: Choose foods with lower acidity to lessen the probability of initiating acid reflux. High-acid meals may irritate the oesophagus and lead to reflux episodes. Opt for fruits like bananas and melons, vegetables like leafy greens, and lean meats like chicken and fish.

**2. Complex carbs**: Emphasize complex carbs that are high in fiber. These meals may help control digestion and minimize excessive pressure on the stomach, minimizing the risk of reflux. Include healthy grains such as oats, quinoa, and brown rice in your diet to enhance digestive health.

**3. Lean Proteins**: Choose lean protein sources to prevent excess fat, which may delay stomach emptying and raise the risk of acid reflux. Opt for lean meats like chicken and turkey, fish, tofu, and lentils.

**4. Healthy Fats**: Incorporate healthy fats while reducing saturated and trans fats. Healthy fats assist general wellness without adding to excessive stomach strain. Include avocados, almonds, seeds, and olive oil in moderation.

**5. Portion Control**: Practice portion control to avoid overeating, which may contribute to increased stomach pressure and induce reflux. Use smaller plates, chew food fully, and be cautious of portion sizes to prevent overindulging.

**6. Avoid Trigger Foods**: Identify and avoid personal trigger foods that increase acid reflux symptoms. These may differ among people. Common trigger foods include spicy meals, citrus fruits, tomatoes, chocolate, and caffeinated drinks. Personal triggers may also include certain meals that people find bothersome.

**7. Meal Timing**: Space out meals and avoid eating close to sleep. Eating too close to bedtime might raise the risk of nocturnal reflux. Aim for at least two to three hours between meals and sleep to allow for healthy digestion.

**8. Hydration with Water**: Stay hydrated with water, but be careful of other liquids that may cause acid reflux, such as citrus juices and fizzy drinks. Drink lots of water throughout the day and restrict acidic or carbonated drinks.

**9. Alkaline Foods**: Include alkaline-forming foods in the diet to possibly neutralize acidity and foster a more alkaline environment in the body. Some alkaline-forming foods include green leafy vegetables, almonds, and some fruits like watermelon.

**10. Mindful Eating**: Practise mindful eating to alleviate stress on the digestive system. Eating in a comfortable atmosphere and paying attention to hunger and fullness signals may significantly improve digestion. Sit down for meals, chew food carefully, and relish the dining experience.

These concepts constitute a basis for an acid reflux diet, giving a comprehensive approach to controlling symptoms and boosting digestive well-being. While these recommendations are based on scientific facts, individual reactions may differ. Consulting with a healthcare practitioner or a qualified dietitian may give individualized counsel to adjust these concepts to specific requirements and tastes.

# CHAPTER 9: SELECTING THE RIGHT FOODS

Selecting the proper foods for acid reflux is a sophisticated and customized process that entails knowing the elements that lead to reflux episodes and making smart dietary decisions. This technique tries to prevent irritation to the oesophagus, control stomach acidity, and enhance overall digestive health. Here's a deep and interesting guidance on how to pick the correct foods for acid reflux:

1. **Low-Acid Fruits**: Choose fruits with reduced acidity to lessen the risk of initiating reflux. High-acid fruits may exacerbate the oesophagus. Opt for bananas, melons, and

pears, which have reduced acidity compared to citrus fruits.

**2. Non-Citrus veggies**: Incorporate non-citrus veggies to give vital nutrients without the acidity that may lead to reflux. Include broccoli, cauliflower, carrots, and leafy greens in your diet for a nutrient-rich and low-acid vegetable variety.

**3. Lean Proteins**: Prioritize lean protein sources to prevent excessive fat consumption, which may delay stomach emptying and lead to reflux. Opt for skinless birds, fish, lean cuts of beef or pig, tofu, and lentils as ideal protein alternatives.

**4. Whole Grains**: Choose whole grains that are rich in fiber to regulate digestion and avoid excessive stomach pressure. Incorporate oats, quinoa, brown rice, and whole-grain bread into your diet for a fiber-rich and digestive-friendly carbohydrate option.

**5. Healthy Fats**: Include healthy fats while reducing saturated and trans fats to enhance general health without adding to reflux. Incorporate avocados, almonds, seeds, and olive oil in moderation to give vital fats without producing undue stomach strain.

**6. Dairy substitutes**: Opt for low-fat or plant-based dairy substitutes to lower fat consumption, particularly if dairy causes reflux symptoms. Choose almond milk, soy milk, or low-fat yogurt as dairy replacements that may be kinder on the digestive system.

**7. Herbs and Spices**: Use herbs and spices to flavor meals without depending on high-acid or spicy components that may cause reflux. Experiment with herbs like basil, oregano, and thyme, and utilize milder spices like ginger and turmeric for taste.

**8. Non-Caffeinated Drinks**: Opt for non-caffeinated drinks to prevent boosting stomach acid production, a typical cause for reflux. Choose water, herbal teas, and non-citrus, non-carbonated liquids to remain hydrated without causing acid reflux.

**9. Alkaline-Forming Foods**: Include alkaline-forming foods in the diet to possibly neutralize acidity and produce a more alkaline environment in the body. Incorporate green leafy vegetables, almonds, and some fruits like watermelon to maintain an alkaline balance.

**10. Portion Control**: Practice portion control to avoid overeating and lessen the danger of excessive stomach pressure. Use smaller plates, eat slowly, and pay attention to hunger and fullness signals to prevent overindulging.

It's vital to remember that individual reactions to various meals may differ. Keeping a food diary may help discover personal trigger foods and adapt dietary choices appropriately. Additionally, talking with a healthcare expert or a certified dietitian may give individualized recommendations based on particular health problems and requirements.

This strategy, based on up-to-date scientific evidence, allows people to make educated dietary choices that correspond with their particular digestive needs and help to successfully acid reflux control.

# CHAPTER 10: FOODS TO AVOID FOR ACID REFLUX

Avoiding certain meals is vital for treating acid reflux, since it may help lessen symptoms and avoid spells of pain. While individual triggers may vary, there are common factors known to worsen acid reflux. Here's a deep and new investigation of foods to avoid for acid reflux, anchored in up-to-date scientific information:

**1. High-Acid Fruits**: Fruits with high acidity may cause acid reflux by raising stomach acidity and irritating the oesophagus. Citrus fruits like oranges, lemons, grapefruits, and tomatoes should be limited or avoided.

**2. Spicy Meals**: Spicy meals may accelerate the production of stomach acid and relax the lower esophageal sphincter (LES), leading to reflux. Chili peppers, spicy sauces, and foods severely seasoned with spices like black pepper and chili powder should be controlled.

**3. Fried and Fatty Meals**: High-fat meals might delay stomach emptying and increase pressure on the LES, encouraging reflux. Avoid fried meals, fatty cuts of meat, full-fat dairy products, and heavy sweets, opting for leaner options.

**4. Carbonated Beverages**: Carbonated beverages may raise stomach pressure and stimulate the release of stomach acid, making them possible causes for acid reflux. Limit or avoid sodas, carbonated water, and fizzy drinks.

**5. Caffeine:** Caffeine promotes acid production and may relax the LES, making it preferable to minimize consumption for people prone to acid reflux. Cut down on coffee, tea, energy drinks, and other caffeinated beverages.

**6. Chocolate**: Chocolate includes chemicals that might relax the LES and may lead to increased acid reflux. Limit chocolate bars, desserts, and cocoa-based items.

**7. Mint and Peppermint**: Mint and peppermint may relax the LES, possibly enabling stomach acid to flow back into the oesophagus. Be cautious with mint-flavored products, peppermint tea, and mint candies.

**8. Onions and Garlic**: Onions and garlic may induce relaxation of the LES and raise stomach acidity, leading to acid reflux. Limit raw onions, garlic, and foods with strong onion or garlic content.

**9. Acidic Condiments**: Condiments with excessive acidity might increase acid reflux symptoms. Vinegar-based dressings, ketchup, mustard, and chili sauces should be used sparingly.

**10. Tomato-Based Goods**: Tomatoes are very acidic and may contribute to increased stomach acidity, making tomato-based goods possible triggers for acid reflux. Limit or avoid tomato sauces, ketchup, and meals with a tomato foundation.

**11. Citrus Juices**: Like entire citrus fruits, citrus juices are very acidic and may irritate the oesophagus. Reduce consumption of orange juice, grapefruit juice, and other citrus-based drinks.

**12. Pepper and Salt**: Excessive usage of salt and pepper might lead to increased stomach acidity. Use salt and pepper in moderation and try alternate spices.

**13. Processed Foods**: Processed foods typically include chemicals and preservatives that might lead to acid reflux symptoms. Minimize intake of processed snacks, canned soups, and ready-made meals.

It's necessary to address dietary adjustments for acid reflux on an individual basis, since causes might differ. Keeping a meal journal to identify particular culprits and speaking with a healthcare expert or a qualified dietitian might give individualized recommendations. This strategy, anchored on up-to-date scientific evidence, helps people to make educated choices regarding their food and successfully manage acid reflux symptoms.

# PART 3

---

# CREATING REFLUX-FRIENDLY MEALS

# CHAPTER 11: BREAKFASTS FOR A HEALTHY START

## 1. Tropical Oatmeal

*Ingredients:*

- 1/2 cup rolled oats
- 1/2 cup unsweetened coconut milk
- 1/2 cup diced fresh pineapple
- 1/2 banana, sliced
- 1 tablespoon unsweetened shredded coconut

**Preparation**:

Cook oats according to package directions. Top with coconut milk, pineapple, banana, and shredded coconut.

**Nutritional information**: 350 calories, 10g protein, 9g fat, 62g carbohydrates, 9g fiber, 20g sugar

**Cooking time**: 10 minutes

## 2. Whole Grain Muffin

*Ingredients*:

- 1 whole grain muffin
- 1 tablespoon almond butter
- 1/2 banana, sliced

**Preparation**:

Toast muffin and spread with almond butter. Top with banana slices.

**Nutritional Information**: 250 calories, 7g protein, 8g fat, 40g carbohydrates, 6g fiber, 12g sugar

**Cooking time**: 5 minutes

# 3. Nutty Breakfast Cereal

*Ingredients*:

- 1/2 cup cooked quinoa
- 1/2 cup unsweetened almond milk
- 1/2 apple, diced
- 1 tablespoon chopped walnuts
- 1 teaspoon honey

**Preparation**:

Combine quinoa, almond milk, apple, walnuts, and honey in a bowl.

**Nutritional Information**: 250 calories, 7g protein, 9g fat, 38g carbohydrates, 6g fiber, 14g sugar

**Cooking time**: 15 minutes

## 4. Boiled Egg

### *Ingredients*

- 1 boiled egg
- 1 slice whole grain bread
- 1/2 avocado, sliced

**Preparation**:

Toast toast and top with sliced avocado. Serve with cooked egg.

**Nutritional Information**: 300 calories, 13g protein, 16g fat, 25g carbohydrates, 9g fiber, 2g sugar

**Cooking time**: 10 minutes

# 5. Breakfast Smoothie

*Ingredients*:

- 1/2 cup frozen mixed berries
- 1/2 banana
- 1/2 cup unsweetened almond milk
- 1/2 cup plain Greek yogurt
- 1 teaspoon honey

**Preparation**:

Combine all ingredients in a blender and mix until smooth.

**Nutritional Information**: 250 calories, 16g protein, 5g fat, 40g carbohydrates, 6g fiber, 25g sugar

**Cooking time**: 5 minutes

# 6. Fruit and Yogurt

*Ingredients*:

- 1/2 cup plain Greek yogurt
- 1/2 cup mixed berries
- 1/2 banana, sliced
- 1 tablespoon chopped walnuts
- 1 teaspoon honey

**Preparation**:

Combine yogurt, berries, banana, walnuts, and honey in a dish.

**Nutritional Information**: 250 calories, 16g protein, 8g fat, 35g carbohydrates, 6g fiber, 20g sugar

**Cooking time**: 5 minutes

# 7. Zucchini Bread

***Ingredients***:

- 1 slice zucchini bread
- 1 tablespoon almond butter
- 1/2 banana, sliced

**Preparation**:

Toast bread and spread with almond butter. Top with banana slices.

**Nutritional Information**: 250 calories, 6g protein, 10g fat, 36g carbohydrates, 2g fiber, 16g sugar

**Cooking time**: 5 minutes

## 8. Savory Crepes

*Ingredients*:

- 1 savory crepe
- 1/2 cup sliced mushrooms
- 1/2 cup baby spinach
- 1/4 cup crumbled feta cheese

**Preparation**:

Heat crepe in a pan. Top with mushrooms, spinach, and feta cheese. Fold the crepe in half.

**Nutritional Information**: 300 calories, 14g protein, 12g fat, 35g carbohydrates, 4g fiber, 6g sugar

**Cooking time**: 10 minutes

# 9. Pear Banana Nut Muffins

***Ingredients***

- 1 cup all-purpose flour
- 1/2 cup whole wheat flour
- 1/2 cup rolled oats
- 1/2 cup chopped walnuts
- 1/2 teaspoon baking soda
- 1/2 teaspoon baking powder
- 1/2 teaspoon salt
- 1/2 teaspoon cinnamon
- 1/4 teaspoon nutmeg
- 1/2 cup unsweetened applesauce
- 1/2 cup mashed ripe banana
- 1/2 cup chopped pear
- 1/4 cup honey
- 1/4 cup canola oil
- 2 eggs

**Preparation**:

1. Preheat oven to 375°F
2. In a large basin, mix together flours, oats, walnuts, baking soda, baking powder, salt, cinnamon, and nutmeg.
3. In a separate bowl, stir together applesauce, banana, pear, honey, oil, and eggs.
4. Add wet ingredients to dry ingredients and whisk until just blended.
5. Divide batter into 12 muffin cups. Bake for 15-20 minutes.

**Nutritional Information**: 180 calories, 10g fat, 20g carbohydrates, 2g fiber, 8g sugar

**Cooking time**: 35 minutes

# 10. Bajra Roti

***Ingredients***:

- 1 cup bajra or black millet, steeped overnight or for 8 hours
- 1 cup yellow moong dal or split beans, cleaned and set aside
- 1/2 tablespoon ghee
- 1 teaspoon cumin seeds
- 1/2 teaspoon finely chopped ginger paste, salt as per taste
- 3/4 cup yogurt or buttermilk
- 2 green chilies, diced

**Preparation**:

1. Heat oil in a kadhai.
2. Add cumin or nigella seeds.
3. Saute until the seeds flutter.

4. Add ginger paste and cook for a few seconds. Add the dal and cook for a minute.

5. Add 2 cups of water and salt.

6. Cover and heat till the dal is done.

7. Add bajra flour and stir thoroughly.

8. Add yogurt or buttermilk and blend thoroughly. Cook for 5-7 minutes.

9. Serve hot with green chiles.

**Nutritional Information**: 200 calories, 8g protein, 4g fat, 35g carbohydrates, 8g fiber, 2g sugar

**Cooking time**: 30 minutes

**Note**: Nutritional information may vary based on the brand and kind of materials used. culinary time may also vary based on the individual's culinary abilities and equipment.

# CHAPTER 12: LUNCH RECIPES THAT SOOTHE ACID REFLUX

## 1.Tuna Salad on Pita

**Ingredients**:

- 1 can of tuna
- 1 whole wheat pita
- 1/2 cup mixed greens
- 1/4 cup sliced cucumber
- 1 tablespoon olive oil
- 1 tablespoon lemon juice

**Preparation**: Mix tuna, mixed greens, cucumber, olive oil, and lemon juice. Stuff the mixture inside the pita.

**Nutritional Information**: Varies depends on components utilized.

**Cooking time**: 10 minutes

## 2. Brown Rice Bowl with Grilled Vegetables and Chicken Breast

*Ingredients*:

- 1 cup cooked brown rice
- 1 cup grilled veggies (e.g., zucchini, carrots, mushrooms)
- 4 ounces grilled chicken breast

**Preparation**:

Combine brown rice, grilled veggies, and grilled chicken breast in a bowl.

**Nutritional Information**: Varies depends on components utilized.

**Cooking time**: 20 minutes

3. **Baked Salmon with Quinoa and Asparagus**

*Ingredients*:

- 4 oz baked salmon
- 1/2 cup cooked quinoa
- 1/2 cup steaming asparagus

**Preparation**:

Serve baked salmon with cooked quinoa and steamed asparagus.

**Nutritional Information**: Varies depends on components utilized.

**Cooking time**: 25 minutes

## 4. Turkey Meatballs with Whole Grain Pasta and Light Basil and Olive Oil Pesto

*Ingredients*:

- 4 turkey meatballs
- 1 cup cooked whole grain spaghetti
- 2 tablespoons light basil and olive oil pesto

*Preparation*:

Serve turkey meatballs over cooked whole grain pasta and mild basil and olive oil pesto.

**Nutritional Information**: Varies according to components utilized.

**Cooking time**: 30 minutes

# 5. Chicken Fried Rice

*Ingredients*:

- 1 cup cooked brown rice
- 4 ounces chopped chicken breast
- 1/2 cup mixed veggies
- 1 egg
- 1 tablespoon low-sodium soy sauce

**Preparation**:

1. Stir-fry chicken, mixed veggies, and egg.
2. Add cooked brown rice and soy sauce.

**Nutritional Information**: Varies depends on components utilized.

**Cooking time**: 20 minutes

# 6. Pea and Basil Buckwheat Risotto

*Ingredients*:

- 1 cup cooked buckwheat
- 1/2 cup peas

- 1/4 cup chopped basil
- 1/4 cup grated Parmesan cheese

**Preparation**: Combine cooked buckwheat, peas, basil, and Parmesan cheese in a pan.

**Nutritional Information**: Varies according to components utilized.

**Cooking time**: 25 minutes

# 7. Honey-Braised Salmon with Couscous and Kale10

*Ingredients*:

- 4 ounces honey-braised salmon
- 1/2 cup cooked couscous
- 1/2 cup sautéed greens

**Preparation**:

Serve honey-braised salmon over cooked couscous and sautéed greens.

**Nutritional Information**: Varies depends on components utilized.

**Cooking time**: 25 minutes

# 8. Turkey and Vegetable Soup

*Ingredients*:

- 1 cup diced turkey
- 1 cup mixed veggies
- 4 cups low-sodium chicken broth

**Preparation**: Simmer diced turkey and mixed veggies in low-sodium chicken broth.

**Nutritional Information**: Varies depends on components utilized.

**Cooking time**: 30 minutes

# 9. Low-Fat Sandwich

*Ingredients*:

- Whole grain bread
- 4 oz lean turkey or chicken breast, lettuce, sliced cucumber, mustard

**Preparation**:

Assemble the sandwich with lean turkey or chicken breast, lettuce, sliced cucumber, and mustard.

**Nutritional Information**: Varies according to components utilized.

**Cooking time**: 10 minutes

# 10. Chicken and Turkey Noodle Soup

*Ingredients*:

- 4 cups low-sodium chicken broth
- 4 ounces diced chicken or turkey

- 1 cup cooked whole grain noodles
- 1 cup mixed veggies

**Preparation**:

Simmer diced chicken or turkey, cooked whole grain noodles, and mixed veggies in low-sodium chicken broth.

**Nutritional Information**: Varies according to components utilized.

**Cooking time**: 30 minutes

**Note**: Nutritional information may vary based on the brand and kind of materials used. culinary time may also vary based on the individual's culinary abilities and equipment.

# CHAPTER 13: DINNER RECIPES FOR DIGESTIVE COMFORT

## 1. Grilled Chicken Breast with Quinoa and Steamed Broccoli

*Ingredients*:

- 2 boneless, skinless chicken breasts
- 1 cup cooked quinoa
- 1 cup steamed broccoli

**Preparation**:

1. Season chicken breasts with salt and pepper, grill until done.
2. Serve over a bed of cooked quinoa with steamed broccoli on the side.

**Nutritional Information**: Approximately 400 calories, 40g protein, 8g fat, 40g carbs, 7g fiber.

**Cooking Time**: 20 minutes.

## 2. Salmon with Asparagus and Sweet Potato Mash

*Ingredients*:

- 2 salmon fillets
- 1 bunch of asparagus
- 2 medium sweet potatoes, mashed

**Preparation**:

1. Bake fish in the oven, roast asparagus.
2. Serve with a side of mashed sweet potatoes.

**Nutritional Information**: Approximately 450 calories, 35g protein, 15g fat, 40g carbs, 8g fiber.

**Cooking Time**: 25 minutes.

## 3. Vegetarian Stir-Fry with Tofu and Brown Rice

*Ingredients*:

- 1 cup firm tofu, cubed
- 2 cups mixed stir-fry veggies (broccoli, bell peppers, snap peas)
- 1 cup cooked brown rice

**Preparation**:

1. Stir-fry tofu and veggies in a non-stick pan.
2. Serve over cooked brown rice.

**Nutritional Information**: Approximately 380 calories, 20g protein, 12g fat, 50g carbs, 8g fiber.

**Cooking Time**: 15 minutes.

## 4. Turkey and Vegetable Skewers with Quinoa

*Ingredients*:

- 1 pound ground turkey
- Assorted veggies (cherry tomatoes, zucchini, bell peppers)
- 1 cup cooked quinoa

**Preparation**:

1. Form turkey into skewers with veggies.
2. Grill until turkey is done, serve with quinoa.

**Nutritional Information**: Approximately 350 calories, 25g protein, 10g fat, 40g carbs, 6g fiber.

**Cooking Time**: 20 minutes.

## 5. Baked Cod with Roasted Brussels Sprouts and Mashed Cauliflower

***Ingredients***:

- 2 cod fillets
- 2 cups Brussels sprouts, halved
- 1 head cauliflower, mashed

**Preparation**:

1. Bake fish in the oven, roast Brussels sprouts.
2. Serve with mashed cauliflower.

**Nutritional Information**: Approximately 320 calories, 30g protein, 8g fat, 35g carbs, 10g fiber.

**Cooking Time**: 25 minutes.

## 6. Pasta with Spinach and Chicken in Tomato Sauce

*Ingredients*:

- 2 cups whole grain pasta
- 1 cup cooked chicken breast, shredded
- 2 cups fresh spinach
- 1 cup tomato sauce (low-acid)

**Preparation**:

1. Cook pasta according to package directions.
2. Combine with shredded chicken, fresh spinach, and tomato sauce.

**Nutritional Information**: Approximately 400 calories, 25g protein, 10g fat, 50g carbs, 8g fiber.

**Cooking Time**: 20 minutes.

## 7. Eggplant and Chicken Casserole with Quinoa

*Ingredients*:

- 1 big eggplant, cut
- 1 cup cooked chicken breast, diced
- 1 cup cooked quinoa
- 1 cup low-acid tomato sauce

**Preparation**:

1. Layer sliced eggplant, chicken, quinoa, and tomato sauce in a baking dish.
2. Bake until the eggplant is soft.

**Nutritional Information**:  Approximately 380 calories, 30g protein, 10g fat, 40g carbs, 10g fiber.

**Cooking Time**: 30 minutes.

## 8. Shrimp and Vegetable Stir-Fry with Brown Rice

*Ingredients*:

- 1 pound shrimp, peeled and deveined
- Assorted stir-fry veggies (broccoli, snow peas, carrots)
- 1 cup cooked brown rice

**Preparation**:

1. Stir-fry shrimp and veggies in a non-stick pan.
2. Serve over cooked brown rice.

**Nutritional Information**:  Approximately 300 calories, 25g protein, 8g fat, 35g carbs, 5g fiber.

**Cooking Time**: 15 minutes.

## 9. Chickpea and Spinach Curry with Quinoa

*Ingredients*:

- 1 can chickpeas, drained and rinsed
- 2 cups fresh spinach
- 1 cup coconut milk
- 1 cup cooked quinoa

**Preparation**:

1. Simmer chickpeas and spinach in coconut milk until cooked through.
2. Serve over cooked quinoa.

**Nutritional Information**: Approximately 380 calories, 15g protein, 15g fat, 45g carbs, 10g fiber.

**Cooking Time**: 20 minutes.

## 10. Lemon Herb Baked Chicken with Mashed Sweet Potatoes

*Ingredients*:
- 2 boneless, skinless chicken breasts
- 1 lemon, juiced
- 1 teaspoon dried herbs (rosemary, thyme)
- 2 medium sweet potatoes, mashed

**Preparation**:
1. Marinate chicken in lemon juice and spices, bake till done.
2. Serve with mashed sweet potatoes.

**Nutritional Information**:  Approximately 350 calories, 30g protein, 5g fat, 40g carbs, 8g fiber.

**Cooking Time**: 25 minutes.


Remember to change amounts and ingredients depending on your unique dietary requirements and tastes. Nutritional information is approximate and may vary depending on the brands and amounts used.

# CHAPTER 14: REFLUX-FRIENDLY SOUP RECIPES

## 1. Chicken and Black-Eyed Pea Soup

***Ingredients***:

- 1 cup black-eyed peas
- 2 cups diced cooked chicken
- 1 cup chopped carrots
- 1 cup chopped celery
- 4 cups low-sodium chicken broth
- 1 teaspoon thyme
- 1 teaspoon basil
- 2 bay leaves
- 1 teaspoon sage

- 1 teaspoon rosemary

**Preparation**:

1. In a big saucepan, mix all ingredients and bring to a boil.
2. Reduce heat and simmer for 30 minutes.

**Nutritional Information**: Varies according to components utilized.

**Cooking time**: 40 minutes

## 2. Chilled Pea Soup with Herbs

*Ingredients*:

- 2 cups frozen peas
- 1 cup low-sodium vegetable broth
- 1/2 cup chopped onions
- 1/4 cup chopped fresh herbs (e.g., mint, parsley)
- 1/2 cup plain Greek yogurt

**Preparation**:

- In a blender, mix peas, vegetable broth, onions, and herbs.
- Blend until smooth.
- Stir in Greek yogurt.
- Chill before serving.

**Nutritional Information**: Varies according to components utilized.

**Cooking time**: 10 minutes

# 3. Chilled Watermelon Soup

*Ingredients*:

- 4 cups cubed watermelon
- 1/4 cup fresh lime juice
- 1 tablespoon honey
- 1/4 cup chopped mint leaves

**Preparation**:

1. In a blender, mix watermelon, lime juice, honey, and mint leaves.
2. Blend until smooth. Chill before serving.

**Nutritional Information**: Varies according to components utilized.

**Cooking time**: 10 minutes

# 4. Classic Potato Soup

*Ingredients*:

- 4 cups peeled and diced potatoes
- 1 cup chopped onions
- 4 cups low-sodium vegetable broth
- 1 cup unsweetened almond milk
- 1/4 cup chopped green onions

**Preparation**:

1. In a large saucepan, mix potatoes, onions, and vegetable broth.

2.  Bring to a boil, then decrease heat and simmer until potatoes are cooked.

3.  Stir in almond milk. Garnish with green onions before serving.

**Nutritional Information**: Varies according to components utilized.

**Cooking time**: 30 minutes

## 5. Cream of Fava Bean Soup

*Ingredients*:

- 2 cups shelled fava beans
- 1 cup chopped onions
- 4 cups low-sodium vegetable broth
- 1/2 cup unsweetened almond milk
- 1/4 cup chopped fresh parsley

**Preparation**:

1. In a large saucepan, mix fava beans, onions, and vegetable broth.
2. Bring to a boil, then decrease heat and simmer until beans are cooked.
3. Stir in almond milk.
4. Garnish with parsley before serving.

**Nutritional Information**: Varies depends on components utilized.

**Cooking time**: 40 minutes

## 6. Eggplant & Garlic Soup

*Ingredients*:

- 2 cups diced eggplant
- 1 cup chopped onions
- 4 cups low-sodium vegetable broth
- 4 cloves roasted garlic
- 1/4 cup chopped fresh basil

**Preparation**:

- In a large saucepan, mix eggplant, onions, and vegetable broth.
- Bring to a boil, then decrease heat and simmer until eggplant is soft.
- Stir in roasted garlic. Garnish with basil before serving.

**Nutritional Information**: Varies depends on components utilized.

**Cooking time**: 30 minutes

## 7. Fish Soup with Yams

*Ingredients*:

- 4 cups low-sodium fish broth
- 1 cup diced yams
- 1 cup chopped onions
- 2 cups flaked white fish

- 1/4 cup chopped cilantro

**Preparation**:

1. In a big saucepan, mix fish broth, yams, and onions.
2. Bring to a boil, then decrease heat and simmer until yams are soft.
3. Add flaked fish and boil until cooked through. Garnish with cilantro before serving.

**Nutritional information**: Varies according to components utilized.

**Cooking time**: 35 minutes

## 8. Iced Cucumber Soup

*Ingredients*:

- 2 cups sliced cucumbers
- 1 cup plain Greek yogurt

- 1/4 cup chopped fresh dill
- 1 tablespoon lemon juice
- 1/4 cup chopped green onions

**Preparation**:

1. In a blender, mix cucumbers, Greek yogurt, dill, and lemon juice.
2. Blend until smooth. Chill before serving. Garnish with green onions.

**Nutritional Information**: Varies according to components utilized.

**Cooking time**: 10 minutes

# 9. Lentil and Chickpea Soup

*Ingredients*:

- 1 cup dry lentils
- 1 cup cooked chickpeas
- 1 cup chopped carrots
- 1 cup chopped celery

- 4 cups low-sodium vegetable broth
- 1 teaspoon cumin
- 1 teaspoon coriander

**Preparation**:

1. In a large saucepan, add lentils, chickpeas, carrots, celery, and vegetable broth.
2. Bring to a boil, then decrease heat and simmer for 40 minutes.

**Nutritional information**: Varies depends on components utilized.

**Cooking time**: 50 minutes

## 10. Lentil Chili

*Ingredients*:

- 1 cup dry lentils
- 1 cup chopped onions
- 1 cup chopped bell peppers
- 4 cups low-sodium vegetable broth

- 1 can diced tomatoes
- 1 tablespoon chili powder
- 1 teaspoon cumin

**Preparation**:

1. In a large saucepan, add lentils, onions, bell peppers, vegetable broth, chopped tomatoes, chili powder, and cumin.
2. Bring to a boil, then decrease heat and simmer for 40 minutes.

**Nutritional Information**:

Varies according to components utilized.

**Cooking time**: 50 minutes

**Note**: Nutritional information may vary based on the brand and kind of materials used. culinary time may also vary based on the individual's culinary abilities and equipment.

# CHAPTER 15: SALAD RECIPES FOR DIGESTIVE HEALTH

## 1. Calm Carrot Salad for Acid Reflux

***Ingredients***:

- 2 cups shredded carrots
- 1/4 cup raisins
- 1/4 cup orange juice
- 1 tablespoon brown sugar
- 1 Tablespoon olive oil
- 1/2 teaspoon dried oregano
- 1/4 teaspoon salt
- Mesclun departs

**Preparation**:

1. In a mixing bowl, combine the raisins, orange juice, brown sugar, olive oil, oregano, and salt together.
2. Let sit for approximately 5 minutes.
3. Pour the dressing over the carrots and stir completely.
4. Season with more salt as required.
5. Serve over mesclun leaves.

**Nutritional information**: 1 serving (677g) has 494 calories, 32g fat, 47g carbs, 6g fiber, 38g sugar, and 4g protein.

**Cooking time**: Not applicable

## 2. Chopped Mediterranean Salad

*Ingredients*:

- 3 cups chopped arugula
- 1/2 cups cooked chicken

- 1 cup quartered cucumbers
- 1/2 cup chopped kalamata olives
- 1/3 cup chopped artichoke hearts

**Dressing**:

- 1 cup fresh basil
- 1/2 cup olive oil
- 2–3 tbsp nutritional yeast
- 2 tbsp raw pine nuts
- 1 tbsp + 1 tsp lemon juice
- 1/2 tsp salt
- 1 tbsp water

**Preparation**:

1. To make the salad, cut arugula, artichokes, olives, and cucumbers.
2. Add to a salad bowl and mix.
3. To prepare the dressing, add fresh basil, raw pine nuts, nutritional yeast, lemon

juice, water, and salt to a food processor or high-speed blender.

4.  Process and carefully add in the olive oil until you have a smooth consistency and the dressing is emulsified.

5.  Drizzle the dressing over the salad and enjoy.

**Nutritional Information**: 1 serving provides 400 calories, 28g fat, 60mg cholesterol, 12g carbs, 4g fiber, 4g sugar, and 25g protein.

**Cooking time**: 30 minutes (for cooking chicken)

Please note that the preparation time for the Calm Carrot Salad is not relevant since it does not entail cooking. Nutritional statistics may vary based on the brand and kind of components used.

## 3. Chicken and Quinoa Salad

*Ingredients*:

- 1 cup cooked quinoa
- 1 cup grilled chicken breast, sliced
- 1 cup cucumber, diced
- 1 cup cherry tomatoes, halved
- 2 tablespoons olive oil
- 1 tablespoon balsamic vinegar

**Preparation**:

1. In a bowl, mix quinoa, chicken, cucumber, and cherry tomatoes.
2. Drizzle with olive oil and balsamic vinegar, mix to blend.

**Nutritional Information**: Approximately 400 calories, 30g protein, 15g fat, 40g carbs, 5g fiber.

**Cooking Time**: 20 minutes (including quinoa and chicken preparation).

# 4. Salmon and Avocado Salad

*Ingredients*:

- 2 cups mixed greens
- 1 grilled salmon fillet, flaked
- 1/2 avocado, sliced
- 1/4 cup chopped red onion
- 2 teaspoons lemon juice

**Preparation**:

1. Arrange mixed greens on a platter, top with flakes salmon, avocado, and red onion.
2. Drizzle with lemon juice.

**Nutritional Information**:

Approximately 350 calories, 25g protein, 20g fat, 20g carbs, 8g fiber.

**Cooking Time**: 15 minutes (including salmon grilling).

## 5. Spinach and Strawberry Salad

*Ingredients*:

- 2 cups fresh spinach
- 1 cup sliced strawberries
- 1/4 cup crumbled feta cheese
- 2 teaspoons balsamic vinaigrette
- 1 tablespoon chopped almond

**Preparation**:

1. Toss spinach, strawberries, and feta in a bowl.
2. Drizzle with balsamic vinaigrette and sprinkle chopped almonds over top.

**Nutritional Information**:

Approximately 250 calories, 8g protein, 15g fat, 25g carbs, 6g fiber.

**Cooking Time**: 0 minutes.

# 6. Quinoa and Vegetable Salad

*Ingredients*:

- 1 cup cooked quinoa
- 1 cup cherry tomatoes, halved
- 1/2 cup cucumber, diced
- 1/4 cup red bell pepper, chopped
- 2 tablespoons olive oil - 1 tablespoon red wine vinegar

**Preparation:**

1. Combine cooked quinoa, cherry tomatoes, cucumber, and red bell pepper in a bowl.
2. Drizzle with olive oil and red wine vinegar, mix to blend.

**Nutritional Information**:

Approximately 300 calories, 7g protein, 15g fat, 35g carbs, 5g fiber.

**Cooking Time**: 20 minutes (including quinoa preparation).

## 7. Tuna and White Bean Salad

***Ingredients***:

- 1 can (5 oz) tuna, drained
- 1 can (15 oz) white beans, drained and rinsed
- 1/2 cup cherry tomatoes, halved
- 1/4 cup red onion, coarsely chopped
- 2 tablespoons olive oil
- 1 tablespoon lemon juice

**Preparation**:

1. In a bowl, add tuna, white beans, cherry tomatoes, and red onion.
2. Drizzle with olive oil and lemon juice, stir gently.

**Nutritional Information**: Approximately 350 calories, 25g protein, 10g fat, 40g carbs, 10g fiber.

**Cooking Time**: 0 minutes.

## 8. Greek Salad with Grilled Shrimp

*Ingredients*:
- 2 cups mixed greens
- 1/2 cup cherry tomatoes, halved
- 1/4 cup cucumber, sliced
- 1/4 cup kalamata olives, pitted
- 1/4 cup feta cheese, crumbled
- 1/2 pound grilled shrimp
- 2 tablespoons olive oil

- 1 tablespoon red wine vinegar

**Preparation**:
- Arrange mixed greens on a platter, top with cherry tomatoes, cucumber, olives, feta, and grilled shrimp.
- Drizzle with olive oil and red wine vinegar.

**Nutritional Information**: Approximately 400 calories, 30g protein, 20g fat, 20g carbs, 5g fiber.

**Cooking Time**: 15 minutes (including shrimp grilling).

## 9. Caprese Salad with Basil Pesto Chicken

***Ingredients***:

- 2 cups cherry tomatoes, halved
- 1/2 cup fresh mozzarella, diced
- 1/4 cup fresh basil leaves
- 1/2 pound grilled chicken breast, sliced
- 2 teaspoons basil pesto
- 1 tablespoon balsamic glaze

**Preparation**:

1. Combine cherry tomatoes, mozzarella, basil, and grilled chicken in a bowl.
2. Drizzle with basil pesto and balsamic glaze, stir gently.

**Nutritional Information**: Approximately 380 calories, 35g protein, 20g fat, 15g carbs, 3g fiber.

**Cooking Time**: 20 minutes (including chicken grilling).


## 10. Mango and Shrimp Salad

*Ingredients*:

- 2 cups mixed greens
- 1/2 cup cooked shrimp, peeled and deveined
- 1/2 mango, diced
- 1/4 cup red bell pepper, chopped
- 2 teaspoons lime juice
- 1 tablespoon olive oil

**Preparation**:

1. Arrange mixed greens on a platter, top with shrimp, mango, and red bell pepper.
2. Drizzle with lime juice and olive oil.

**Nutritional Information**: Approximately 300 calories, 20g protein, 10g fat, 30g carbs, 5g fiber.

**Cooking Time**: 10 minutes (including shrimp preparation).

## 11. Cucumber and Chickpea Salad

*Ingredients*:

- 2 cucumbers, sliced
- 1 can (15 oz) chickpeas, drained and rinsed
- 1/4 cup red onion, coarsely chopped
- 1/4 cup fresh dill, chopped
- 2 tablespoons olive oil
- 1 tablespoon white wine vinegar

**Preparation**:

1. Combine cucumber, chickpeas, red onion, and fresh dill in a bowl.

2. Drizzle with olive oil and white wine vinegar, stir gently.

**Nutritional Information**: Approximately 250 calories, 8g protein, 10g fat, 35g carbs, 8g fiber.

**Cooking Time**: 0 minutes.

## 12. Turkey and Cranberry Salad

*Ingredients*:

- 2 cups mixed greens
- 1/2 cup cooked turkey breast, sliced
- 1/4 cup dried cranberries
- 1/4 cup walnuts, chopped
- 2 teaspoons cranberry vinaigrette dressing

**Preparation**:

1. Arrange mixed greens on a platter, top with turkey, dried cranberries, and walnuts.
2. Drizzle with cranberry vinaigrette dressing.

**Nutritional Information**: Approximately 320 calories, 20g protein, 15g fat, 30g carbs, 5g fiber.

**Cooking Time**: 0 minutes.

Remember to change amounts and ingredients depending on your unique dietary requirements and tastes. Nutritional information is approximate and may vary depending on the brands and amounts utilized.

# CHAPTER 16: SOOTHING SMOOTHIE RECIPES

---

## 1. Pineapple Banana Smoothie

*Ingredients*:

- 1/2 cups fresh pineapple, chopped
- 1 banana
- 1/2 cup Greek yogurt
- 1/2 cup ice
- 1/2 cup pineapple juice or water

**Preparation**:

1. Add all of the ingredients (pineapple, banana, yogurt, ice, and juice) to a blender and process until it reaches a smoothie consistency.

2. Pour and enjoy!

## 2. Banana Ginger Energy Smoothie

*Ingredients*:

- 1 banana
- 1/2 inch fresh ginger, peeled
- 1 cup unsweetened almond milk
- 1 tsp flax seeds

**Preparation**:

1. Combine the banana, ginger, almond milk, and flaxseeds in a blender.
2. Blend until smooth and creamy.
3. Serve and enjoy!

## 3. Creamy Banana Smoothie

*Ingredients*:

- 2 bananas frozen
- ½ cup vegan yogurt plain
- 1 cup cashew milk
- 1 serving collagen powder or 1 serving homemade protein powder
- 1 tsp vanilla extract

**Instructions:**

1. Blend all ingredients until smooth
2. Pour into your favorite glass and enjoy!

**Notes:** To make this smoothie vegan, switch 1 scoop of collagen powder with 1 serve of homemade protein powder. To minimize the natural fruit sugars, add 1/4 avocado and 1 banana

You may swap in any flavor of yogurt, but select one that's plain or with little sugar

The cashews may be changed for almonds or oats

The cashew milk may be substituted out for the dairy-free milk of your choosing

## Nutrition Information

Serving: 16oz, Calories: 364 kcal, Carbohydrates: 61g, Protein: 18g, Fat: 7g, Saturated Fat: 3g, Polyunsaturated Fat: 1g, Monounsaturated Fat: 2g, Cholesterol: 16mg, Sodium: 255mg, Potassium: 1041 mg, Fiber: 6g, Sugar: 35g, Vitamin A: 272IU, Vitamin C: 21mg, Calcium: 160mg, Iron: 1mg

# 4. Creamy Pumpkin Smoothie

## *Ingredients*

- 1 cup spinach
- 1 cup almond milk unsweetened
- ½ cup pumpkin puree unsweetened
- ½ banana frozen
- ½ cup mango frozen
- 1 tsp pumpkin spice
- ½ tsp vanilla extract
- 1 serving homemade protein powder optional

## Instructions

1. Blend spinach and almond milk until smooth.
2. Add additional ingredients and mix again until smooth.

**Notes:**

1. Feel free to use fresh pumpkin puree instead of canned.

2. Swap the spinach with the leafy greens of your choice.

3. To minimize the natural fruit sugar, switch the mango with 1/4 an avocado or 1/2 cup cauliflower.

4. If you can't locate pumpkin pie spice, try my own blend: 1/4 cup ground cinnamon, 3 tablespoons ground ginger, 1 teaspoon ground nutmeg, 1/2 teaspoon each ground cloves, ground allspice and ground cardamom.

5. You can store this in a jar with your other spices and use in smoothies, cookies, pancakes, and more!

6. Add in plant-based protein powder to convert this smoothie into a meal replacement.

7.  Swap almond milk with the unsweetened, dairy-free milk of your choice.

**Nutritional Information:**

Calories: 172 kcal, Carbohydrates: 33g, Protein: 4g, Fat: 4g, Saturated Fat: 1g, Polyunsaturated Fat: 2g, Monounsaturated Fat: 2g, Sodium: 352mg, Potassium: 731mg, Fiber: 5g, Sugar: 21g, Vitamin A: 8686IU, Vitamin C: 49mg, Calcium: 368mg, Iron: 2mg

# 5. Alkaline Smoothie

*Ingredients:*

- ½ cup spinach
- ½ cup dinosaur kale also called lacinato kale
- 1 cup Jovē Alkaline water
- 1 lime
- ½ cucumber

- 1 cup peach frozen
- 1 serving homemade protein powder optional

## Instructions

1. Blend leafy greens with Jovē Alkaline water till smooth.
2. Add additional ingredients and whisk until smooth.

## Notes:

1. Use at least one frozen ingredient for a pleasantly cool smoothie.
2. Use spinach or kale if preferred, or any leafy green of your choosing.
3. Swap alkaline water with filtered water or coconut water.
4. Peaches give this smoothie a somewhat sweet flavor while also making it incredibly creamy.

**Nutritional Information:**

Calories: 107 kcal, Carbohydrates: 26g, Protein: 4g, Fat: 1g, Saturated Fat: 1g, Polyunsaturated Fat: 1g, Monounsaturated Fat: 1g, Sodium: 23 mg, Potassium: 700mg, Fiber: 6g, Sugar: 16g, Vitamin A: 3099IU, Vitamin C: 51mg, Calcium: 116 mg, Iron: 2mg

# 6. Banana Oatmeal Smoothie

*Ingredients*

- ½ cup rolled oats
- 1 cup coconut milk
- 1 banana frozen
- ½ tsp ground cinnamon
- 1 tsp vanilla extract
- ½ tsp maple syrup optional
- 1 serving homemade protein powder optional

## Instructions

- Place all items in a blender.
- Blend until smooth and creamy.
- Pour into a glass and drink immediately.

## Notes:

1. If the smoothie is too thick, add a bit of additional coconut milk and mix again. For a thicker smoothie, add another 1/2 frozen banana.
2. With coconut milk, you may pick canned or refrigerated. Look for light options if you're managing your calories. Or create your own coconut milk right here.
3. Use at least 1 frozen fruit for a pleasantly chilled smoothie.

**Nutritional Information**

Calories: 449 kcal, Carbohydrates: 65g, Protein: 7g, Fat: 16g, Saturated Fat: 14g, Polyunsaturated Fat: 1g, Monounsaturated Fat: 1g, Sodium: 171mg, Potassium: 587 mg, Fiber: 8g, Sugar: 17g, Vitamin A: 78IU, Vitamin C: 10mg, Calcium: 41mg, Iron: 2mg

# CHAPTER 17: DESSERTS RECIPES WITHOUT THE BURN

---

## 1. Coconut & Cacao Loaf

*Ingredients*:

- 1 1/2 cups coconut flour
- 1/2 cup cacao powder
- 1/2 cup coconut oil
- 1/2 cup maple syrup
- 1 tsp vanilla extract
- 1/2 tsp baking soda
- 1/2 tsp salt
- 4 eggs

**Preparation**:

1. Preheat the oven to 350°F.
2. Grease a loaf pan with coconut oil.
3. In a bowl, combine the coconut flour, cacao powder, baking soda, and salt.
4. In another dish, mix together the coconut oil, maple syrup, vanilla extract, and eggs.
5. Combine the wet and dry ingredients and stir until completely incorporated.
6. Pour the batter into the loaf pan and bake for 45-50 minutes.

**Cooking time**: 45-50 minutes

## 2. Paleo Vanilla Sponge Cake

*Ingredients*:

- 2 cups almond flour
- 1/2 cup coconut flour
- 1/2 cup coconut sugar

- 1/2 cup coconut oil

- 4 eggs

- 1 tsp vanilla extract

- 1/2 tsp baking soda

- 1/4 tsp salt

**Preparation**:

1. Preheat the oven to 350°F.

2. Grease a cake pan with coconut oil.

3. In a bowl, combine the almond flour, coconut flour, coconut sugar, baking soda, and salt.

4. In another dish, mix together the coconut oil, eggs, and vanilla extract.

5. Combine the wet and dry ingredients and stir until completely incorporated.

6. Pour the batter into the cake pan and bake for 25-30 minutes.

**Cooking time**: 25-30 minutes

### 3. Cherry & Almond Clafoutis

*Ingredients*:

- 1 pound cherries, pitted
- 1/2 cup almond flour
- 1/4 cup coconut sugar
- 1 cup almond milk
- 4 eggs
- 1 tsp vanilla extract
- 1/4 tsp salt

**Preparation**:

1. Preheat the oven to 350°F.
2. Grease a baking dish with coconut oil.
3. Arrange the cherries in the baking dish.
4. In a bowl, mix together the almond flour, coconut sugar, almond milk, eggs, vanilla essence, and salt.

5. Pour the mixture over the cherries and bake for 35-40 minutes.

**Cooking time**: 35-40 minutes

# 4. Mandarin & Almond Cake

*Ingredients*:

- 1/2 cups almond flour
- 1/2 cup coconut sugar
- 1/4 cup coconut oil
- 4 eggs
- 1/4 cup mandarin juice
- 1 tsp mandarin zest
- 1/2 tsp baking soda
- 1/4 tsp salt

**Preparation**:

1. Preheat the oven to 350°F.
2. Grease a cake pan with coconut oil.

3.  In a bowl, combine the almond flour,
    coconut sugar, baking soda, and salt.

4.  In another dish, mix together the coconut
    oil, eggs, mandarin juice, and mandarin
    zest.

5.  Combine the wet and dry ingredients and
    stir until completely incorporated.

6.  Pour the batter into the cake pan and bake
    for 25-30 minutes.

**Cooking time**: 25-30 minutes

## 5. Paleo Chocolate Chip Cookies

*Ingredients*:

- 2 cups almond flour
- 1/4 cup coconut oil
- 1/4 cup maple syrup
- 1 tsp vanilla extract
- 1/2 tsp baking soda

- 1/4 tsp salt
- 1/2 cup dark chocolate chips

**Preparation**:

1. Preheat the oven to 350°F.
2. Line a baking sheet with parchment paper.
3. In a bowl, combine the almond flour, baking soda, and salt.
4. In another dish, mix together the coconut oil, maple syrup, and vanilla extract.
5. Combine the wet and dry ingredients and stir until completely incorporated.
6. Fold in the chocolate chips.
7. Drop spoonfuls of dough onto the baking sheet and bake for 10-12 minutes.

**Cooking time**: 10-12 minutes

# CHAPTER 18: SNACKS RECIPES

## 1. Yogurt Parfait with Berries

*Ingredients*:

- 1 cup plain Greek yogurt
- 1/2 cup mixed berries (blueberries, strawberries)
- 2 tablespoons honey
- 1/4 cup granola (low-fat)

**Preparation**:

1. Layer Greek yogurt, mixed berries, and granola in a glass.
2. Drizzle with honey.

**Nutritional Information**: Approximately 250 calories, 15g protein, 5g fat, 35g carbs, 5g fiber.

**Preparation Time**: 5 minutes.

## 2. Baked Apple Chips

***Ingredients***:

- 2 apples, finely sliced
- 1 teaspoon cinnamon
- 1 tablespoon honey (optional)

**Preparation**:

1. Preheat the oven to 200°F (93°C).
2. Toss apple slices with cinnamon and put on a baking pan.
3. Bake for 2-3 hours until crisp.

**Nutritional Information**: Approximately 150 calories, 1g protein, 0g fat, 40g carbs, 6g fiber.

**Cooking Time**: 2-3 hours.

## 3. Vegetable Sticks with Hummus

*Ingredients*:

- 1 cup baby carrots
- 1 cup cucumber, sliced
- 1 cup bell pepper strips
- 1/2 cup hummus

**Preparation**:

1. Arrange veggie sticks on a platter.
2. Serve with hummus for dipping.

**Nutritional Information**: Approximately 200 calories, 5g protein, 10g fat, 25g carbs, 8g fiber.

**Preparation Time**: 5 minutes.

## 4. Almond Butter and Banana Rice Cakes

*Ingredients*:

- 2 rice cakes
- 2 tablespoons almond butter
- 1 banana, sliced
- Preparation:
- Spread almond butter on rice cakes.
- Top with banana slices.

**Nutritional Information**: Approximately 250 calories, 7g protein, 12g fat, 30g carbs, 4g fiber.

**Preparation Time**: 5 minutes.

# 5. Edamame Salad

*Ingredients*:

- 1 cup edamame, steamed
- 1/2 cup cherry tomatoes, halved
- 1/4 cup red onion, finely chopped
- 2 tablespoons olive oil
- 1 tablespoon lemon juice

**Preparation**:

1. Combine edamame, cherry tomatoes, and red onion in a bowl.
2. Drizzle with olive oil and lemon juice, stir gently.

**Nutritional Information**: Approximately 180 calories, 12g protein, 10g fat, 15g carbs, 5g fiber.

**Preparation Time**: 10 minutes.

# 6. Rice Cake with Avocado and Smoked Salmon

*Ingredients*

- 2 rice cakes
- 1/2 avocado, mashed
- 2 ounces smoked salmon
- 1 tablespoon capers

**Preparation**:

1. Spread mashed avocado on rice cakes.
2. Top with smoked salmon and capers.

**Nutritional Information**: Approximately 300 calories, 15g protein, 15g fat, 25g carbs, 4g fiber.

**Preparation Time**: 5 minutes.

## 7. Banana and Almond Smoothie

*Ingredients*:

- 1 banana
- 1 cup almond milk (unsweetened)
- 1 tablespoon almond butter
- Ice cubes (optional)

**Preparation**:

1. Blend banana, almond milk, and almond butter until smooth.
2. Add ice cubes as desired.

**Nutritional Information**: Approximately 200 calories, 5g protein, 10g fat, 25g carbs, 5g fiber.

**Preparation Time**: 5 minutes.

# 8. Cottage Cheese with Pineapple

*Ingredients*:

- 1/2 cup low-fat cottage cheese
- 1/2 cup fresh pineapple chunks

**Preparation**:

1. Combine cottage cheese and pineapple in a bowl.
2. Mix thoroughly before serving.

**Nutritional Information**: Approximately 150 calories, 15g protein, 2g fat, 20g carbs, 2g fiber.

**Preparation Time**: 5 minutes.

# 9. Turkey and Cheese Roll-Ups

*Ingredients*:

- 4 slices turkey breast
- 2 slices low-fat cheese
- 1/2 cucumber, divided into thin strips

**Preparation**:

1. Place a piece of cheese on each turkey slice, add cucumber strips.
2. Roll up firmly and fasten with toothpicks.

**Nutritional Information**: Approximately 200 calories, 20g protein, 8g fat, 10g carbs, 2g fiber.

**Preparation Time**: 5 minutes.

# 10. Whole Grain Crackers with Tuna Salad

*Ingredients*:

- 1 can (5 ounce) tuna , drained
- 1/4 cup Greek yogurt (plain, unsweetened)
- 1 tablespoon lemon juice
- 1/4 cup celery, finely chopped
- Whole grain crackers

**Preparation**:

1. In a bowl, combine tuna, Greek yogurt, lemon juice, and celery.
2. Serve with whole grain crackers.

**Nutritional Information**: Approximately 250 calories, 20g protein, 8g fat, 25g carbs, 4g fiber.

**Preparation Time**: 10 minutes.

Remember to change amounts and ingredients depending on your unique dietary requirements and tastes. Nutritional information is approximate and may vary depending on the brands and amounts utilized.

# CHAPTER 19: COOKING TECHNIQUES FOR A REFLUX-FRIENDLY KITCHEN

Creating a reflux-friendly kitchen entails not just choosing the proper products but also adopting cooking procedures that reduce the chance of provoking acid reflux symptoms. By implementing particular approaches into your cooking regimen, you may enjoy rich and fulfilling meals without sacrificing your digestive health.

**1. Steam, Don't Fry**: Opting for steaming over frying is a key strategy that lowers the use of additional oils and minimizes the creation of chemicals that may irritate the oesophagus. Steaming veggies, meats, and grains helps maintain nutrients and natural tastes without adding additional fat.

**2. Grill with Precision**: Grilling is a popular cooking technique that gives a smoky taste to dishes. However, it's necessary to grill with precision to prevent charring, which may create chemicals linked with increased acidity. Keep the grill temperature reasonable, and choose lean meats or veggies to limit the chance of flare-ups.

**3. Poach for Gentleness**: Poaching is a mild cooking method that includes simmering food in liquid. This approach is particularly good for proteins like fish or poultry. Poaching helps maintain moisture without the need for extra fats, adding to a lighter and more digestible meal.

**4. Choose Low-Fat Cooking Methods**: Opting for low-fat cooking techniques such as baking, broiling, or sautéing with little oil will drastically decrease the fat level in your food. High-fat meals might relax the lower esophageal sphincter, causing acid reflux. Using non-stick cookware and integrating herbs and spices for flavor may boost taste without depending on additional oil.

**5. Utilize Aromatics Wisely**: Aromatics like garlic and onions provide dimension to many foods, but they also trigger acid reflux. To still enjoy their tastes, try using infused oils or boiling them completely to break down chemicals that may cause discomfort. Alternatively, exploring herbs like basil, oregano, and ginger may deliver powerful tastes without the danger for reflux.

**6. Acidic Ingredients in Moderation**: While acidic foods like tomatoes may be difficult for reflux patients, utilizing them in moderation and applying cooking procedures to neutralize acidity might make them more acceptable. Slow-roasting tomatoes or adding a bit of baking powder might help balance tastes without creating pain.

**7. Prioritize Lean Proteins**: Opting for lean proteins, such as chicken, fish, and plant-based sources like tofu, minimizes the fat amount in your meals. Excess fat might delay stomach emptying and increase the incidence of acid reflux. Combining lean proteins with reflux-friendly cooking procedures delivers a delicious and digestible protein supply.

**8. Mindful Seasoning**: Seasoning plays a key function in generating delectable food. However, those with acid reflux should be careful with very spicy or strongly seasoned foods. Experimenting with gentler options like fresh herbs, citrus zest, and light spices may increase flavor without creating pain.

**9. Meal Timing and Portion Control**: Beyond cooking procedures, paying attention to meal scheduling and amount management may dramatically improve GERD symptoms. Eating smaller, more frequent meals and avoiding big meals close to sleep might help reduce extra strain on the stomach, lowering the incidence of acid reflux.

**10. Experiment and Listen to Your Body**: Ultimately, the secret to designing a reflux-friendly kitchen rests in experimenting and paying attention to your body's cues. Each person may have distinct triggers, and maintaining a food diary might assist discover particular items or cooking techniques that lead to pain. Adjusting recipes depending on personal tolerance gives a tailored approach to reflux-friendly cooking.

Incorporating these cooking methods into your culinary arsenal not only fosters a reflux-friendly kitchen but also offers up a world of various and pleasurable food possibilities. By employing a conscious and educated approach to cooking, people may experience great tastes without sacrificing their digestive well-being.

# PART 4

---

# LIFESTYLE AND DIETARY HABITS

# CHAPTER 20: EATING HABITS FOR ACID REFLUX RELIEF

Relief from acid reflux frequently starts with establishing mindful eating habits that promote intestinal health. By making conscious choices in your regular meals and snacks, you may reduce symptoms and create a more pleasant eating experience. Let's study innovative and detailed eating habits that haven't been thoroughly covered elsewhere, backed by up-to-date scientific evidence.

**1. Chew Thoroughly and Mindfully**: Scientifically called as mastication, the act of completely chewing food is a key but frequently ignored part of digestive health. Chewing breaks down food into tiny bits, assisting the digestive enzymes in the stomach. This lessens the burden on the stomach and decreases the chances of indigestion and acid reflux. Mindful chewing also increases improved sense of fullness, limiting overeating, and lowering strain on the lower esophageal sphincter (LES).

**2. Optimize Meal Composition**: Consider the content of your meals, concentrating on a balance of macronutrients - proteins, carbs, and fats. Including fiber-rich meals, such as fruits, vegetables, and whole grains, helps improve digestion and regular bowel movements. Fiber may also help to weight control, minimizing the danger of increased strain on the stomach that can lead to acid reflux.

**3. Mind The Time**: Eating habits extend beyond food selections to incorporate meal time.

Aim for regular, spaced-out meals rather than big, occasional ones. Allow at least two to three hours between supper and bedtime to ensure that the stomach has ample time to empty before laying down. This approach may considerably lower the incidence of acid reflux throughout the night.

**4. Experiment with Fermented Foods**: Incorporating fermented foods into your diet offers helpful probiotics, maintaining a healthy gut microbiota. Probiotics contribute to the balance of healthy bacteria in the digestive tract, possibly relieving symptoms of acid reflux. Yogurt, kefir, sauerkraut, and kimchi are examples of fermented foods that may be included in meals or enjoyed as snacks.

**5. Consider Alkaline Foods**: While the notion of alkaline diets for acid reflux alleviation has received prominence, it's vital to approach it with a nuanced viewpoint. Some studies show that eating more alkaline meals, such as some fruits and vegetables, may have a moderate influence on lowering acidity in the stomach. However, individual reactions might differ, and moderation is crucial.

**6. Hydrate Mindfully**: While being hydrated is vital for general health, the manner you drink fluids might impact acid reflux symptoms. Drinking excessive quantities of drink with meals might dilute stomach acid, thereby impairing digestion. Instead, try drinking water between meals and being appropriately hydrated throughout the day to maintain normal digestive function.

**7. Diversify Protein Sources**: Protein is a vital component of a well-rounded diet, but the source of protein matters for acid reflux patients. Consider including lean protein sources, such as chicken, fish, tofu, and lentils, into your meals. Limiting the consumption of high-fat and processed meats minimizes the chance of delayed stomach emptying and consequent reflux.

**8. Mindful Beverage Choices**: Beyond lunch, beverage choices have a key influence in treating acid reflux. Opt for non-acidic drinks, such as herbal teas, water, or almond milk. Limiting or eliminating caffeinated and carbonated beverages may help prevent excess acid production and limit irritation of the oesophagus.

**9. Gentle Cooking Methods**: The manner food is cooked may affect its digestion. Choose moderate cooking techniques like steaming, baking, or poaching instead than frying or grilling with excessive heat. These strategies assist in retaining nutrients while lowering the probability of creating substances that may lead to acid reflux.

**10. Embrace a Personalized Approach**: Acid reflux causes might differ across people, making it necessary to take a tailored approach to eating habits. Keep a food journal to discover particular foods or eating habits that connect with symptoms. Experiment with modifications to see what works best for your individual digestive system.

Treatment from acid reflux includes a comprehensive approach to eating habits that goes beyond merely avoiding trigger foods. By including attentive chewing, improving meal composition, and addressing the scheduling of meals, people may create a more supportive environment for digestive health. Additionally, experimenting with fermented foods, alkaline alternatives, and varied protein sources adds depth to the toolset for treating acid reflux symptoms. Remember that individual reactions may vary, and engaging with healthcare experts or qualified dietitians may give individualized counsel for successful acid reflux treatment.

# CHAPTER 21: INCORPORATING EXERCISE FOR DIGESTIVE HEALTH

In the field of digestive health, exercise is emerging as a potent and sometimes underappreciated ally, with advantages that extend beyond weight control and cardiovascular fitness. While the association between exercise and acid reflux may not be immediately evident, current research results shed light on the tremendous influence physical activity may have on digestive well-being.

**1. Understanding the Link**: Scientific study reveals that regular exercise might favorably affect numerous aspects related with acid reflux.

Exercise helps to maintain a healthy body weight, minimizing the possibility of increased abdominal pressure that may lead to the backward passage of stomach acid into the oesophagus. Additionally, physical exercise may improve more effective digestion by promoting regular bowel movements and reducing constipation, a significant factor to acid reflux.

**2. Aerobic Exercise and Acid Reflux**: Aerobic or cardiovascular activity, such as brisk walking, jogging, or cycling, has been demonstrated to have special advantages for acid reflux patients. Engaging in aerobic exercises helps maintain a healthy body weight, minimizing the risk of belly obesity, a key role in the development of acid reflux symptoms. Moreover, aerobic exercise may strengthen the function of the lower esophageal sphincter (LES), the muscle valve that separates the stomach from the oesophagus, hence avoiding acid reflux episodes.

**3. Yoga and Digestive Wellness**: The practice of yoga, with its focus on gentle movements, regulated breathing, and relaxation methods, has attracted recognition for its potential in boosting digestive health. Certain yoga postures, such as the "Cat-Cow" stretch and "Child's Pose," might help ease intestinal distress by stretching and massaging the abdominal organs. Moreover, the contemplative components of yoga may aid to stress reduction, a recognized cause for acid reflux.

**4. Core Strengthening Exercises**: A strong core offers crucial support for the digestive organs and adds to improved posture. Pilates and core-strengthening activities, when done properly, may help stabilize the abdomen area and alleviate strain on the LES. These exercises enhance total core strength, perhaps benefiting in the avoidance of acid reflux attacks.

**5. Timing Matters**: While exercise is usually excellent for digestive health, the time of physical activity surrounding meals might affect its effect on acid reflux. Exercising too soon after eating may raise the chance of reflux symptoms. It's advised to leave at least two to three hours between meals and hard activity to minimize unnecessary strain on the stomach and LES.

**6. Posture and Digestion**: Maintaining excellent posture is a simple but effective method to improve digestive health. Poor posture may add to intra-abdominal pressure, possibly leading to acid reflux. Whether sitting or standing, having an upright posture helps minimize undue compression of the stomach and lowers the probability of stomach acid leaking back into the oesophagus.

**7. Hydration and Exercise**: Staying appropriately hydrated is crucial for general health and has a role in digestive well-being. During exercise, especially aerobic activity, keeping sufficient hydration helps avoid dehydration, which may lead to constipation—a recognized contributor in acid reflux. Sipping water throughout the day and keeping hydrated throughout exercises aids good digestion.

**8. Individualized Approach**: It's vital to note that the association between exercise and acid reflux might differ across people. While some may find comfort via cardiovascular activities, others may benefit from low-impact workouts or specialized yoga postures. Adopting a tailored approach to exercise that matches with personal preferences and health circumstances guarantees a sustained and successful plan for digestive health.

Adding exercise into one's routine is a comprehensive and unique way to maintain digestive health and control acid reflux symptoms. Scientific research emphasizes the multiple advantages of exercise, from sustaining a healthy body weight to boosting the function of the LES and encouraging effective digestion. Whether via cardiovascular activities, yoga, core-strengthening exercises, or keeping excellent posture, people may adjust their exercise routines to meet their particular digestive demands. As with any health-related activity, consultation with healthcare specialists or fitness experts may give individualized assistance for incorporating exercise into a complete acid reflux treatment strategy.

# CHAPTER 22: STRESS MANAGEMENT TECHNIQUES

Effectively controlling stress is not only excellent for emotional well-being but may also play a vital role in relieving symptoms of acid reflux. Recent scientific studies underline the deep relationship between stress and gastrointestinal health, making stress management strategies a unique and vital part of acid reflux therapy.

**1. Understanding the Gut-Brain Axis**: The gut-brain axis is a bidirectional communication network between the gastrointestinal system and the brain. Scientific study has highlighted the influence of stress on gut function, impacting the development and severity of different digestive illnesses, including acid reflux. Stress stimulates the sympathetic nervous system, resulting in physiological changes that might impair the motility of the digestive tract and enhance the impression of pain.

**2. Mindfulness Meditation**: Mindfulness meditation has earned a reputation for its capacity to alleviate stress and increase general well-being. Studies have demonstrated that mindfulness techniques, which entail paying attention to the present moment without judgement, might favorably affect gastrointestinal symptoms, including acid reflux. Mindful breathing and guided meditation may help people manage stress and develop a more harmonious gut-brain link.

**3. Progressive Muscle Relaxation (PMR):** Progressive Muscle Relaxation is a stress management method that includes repeatedly tensing and then releasing various muscle groups. This procedure helps remove bodily tension and promotes a mood of relaxation. By frequently practicing PMR, people may notice a decrease in stress levels, possibly decreasing the influence of stress on acid reflux symptoms.

**4. Yoga for Stress Relief**: Yoga, with its blend of physical postures, regulated breathing, and meditation, provides a complete approach to stress management. Certain yoga postures, such as child's pose and corpse pose, encourage relaxation and might be especially good for persons living with acid reflux. Scientific studies have proved the favorable benefits of yoga on lowering stress and enhancing gastrointestinal function.

**5. Biofeedback Therapy**: Biofeedback is a therapeutic practice that helps patients achieve awareness and control over physiological processes. In the context of acid reflux and stress management, biofeedback may be used to monitor and modulate muscular tension, heart rate, and other stress-related parameters. Learning to manage these physiological reactions may lead to a more balanced intestinal environment.

**6. Cognitive Behavioral Therapy (CBT):** Cognitive Behavioral Therapy is a well-established psychological technique that tackles cognitive patterns and behaviors related to stress. In the setting of acid reflux, CBT may help patients recognize and confront stress-inducing ideas, developing improved coping skills. Scientific studies indicate the usefulness of CBT in lowering both stress and gastrointestinal problems.

**7. Aromatherapy**: Aromatherapy is the use of essential oils to enhance relaxation and relieve stress. Certain smells, such as lavender and peppermint, have been associated with soothing effects. Incorporating aromatherapy into stress management strategies, such as diffusing essential oils or utilizing them during relaxation exercises, may produce a calming atmosphere that benefits digestive health.

**8. Social Support and Connection**: Social support is an important part in stress management. Engaging in pleasant social interactions and keeping a solid support system may help buffer the effect of stress on acid reflux. Sharing problems, seeking advice, and developing relationships with people contribute to emotional well-being, possibly lowering the physiological impacts of stress on the gastrointestinal system.

**9. Regular Exercise for Stress Reduction**: Physical exercise is a well-established stress management strategy. Regular exercise has been demonstrated to lower stress hormones and boost the production of endorphins, the body's natural mood enhancers. Engaging in activities such as walking, running, or yoga may be especially useful in minimizing the influence of stress on acid reflux.

**10. Balanced Diet**: Proper diet is crucial to stress management and digestive health. Consuming a well-balanced diet that contains nutrient-dense foods enhances general well-being. Nutrients like omega-3 fatty acids, present in fish and flaxseeds, have been connected with stress reduction and may lead to a healthy gut environment.

The integration of stress management approaches into acid reflux therapy constitutes an innovative and complete approach to gastrointestinal health. The scientific study of the gut-brain axis reveals the complicated connection between stress and digestive function. By adopting mindfulness practices, relaxation methods, and social support, people may successfully handle stresses that may lead to acid reflux symptoms. These measures not only boost mental well-being but also create a more suitable atmosphere for digestive health. As usual, speaking with healthcare specialists may give specific counsel for those seeking unique stress management solutions.

# PART 5

# RECIPES FOR SPECIAL

# OCCASIONS

# CHAPTER 24: REFLUX-FRIENDLY HOLIDAY FEASTS

## 1. Herb-Roasted Turkey

*Ingredients*:

- 1 whole turkey (10-12 lbs)
- Fresh herbs (rosemary, thyme, sage)
- Olive oil
- Salt and pepper to taste

**Preparation**:

1. Preheat the oven to 325°F (163°C).
2. Rinse and pat dry the turkey.
3. Rub the turkey with olive oil, fresh herbs, salt, and pepper.

4. Roast until the internal temperature reaches 165°F (74°C).

## 2. Mashed Sweet Potatoes

*Ingredients*:

- 4 medium sweet potatoes, peeled and cubed
- 2 tablespoons unsalted butter
- 1/4 cup almond milk
- Salt and cinnamon to taste

**Preparation**:

1. Boil sweet potatoes till soft.
2. Mash with butter, almond milk, salt, and a touch of cinnamon.

# 3. Quinoa and Cranberry Salad

*Ingredients*:

- 1 cup quinoa, cooked
- 1/2 cup dried cranberries
- 1/4 cup chopped parsley
- 1/4 cup chopped almonds
- Olive oil and lemon dressing

**Preparation**:

1. Mix cooked quinoa, cranberries, parsley, and almonds.
2. Drizzle with olive oil and lemon dressing.

# 4. Green Bean Almondine

*Ingredients*:

- 1 pound fresh green beans, trimmed
- 2 tablespoons slivered almonds
- 2 tablespoons olive oil
- Lemon zest

- Salt and pepper to taste

**Preparation**:
- Blanch green beans in boiling water, then chill in cold water.
- Sauté almonds in olive oil until golden. Add green beans, lemon zest, salt, and pepper.

## 5. Roasted Brussels Sprouts

*Ingredients*:
- 1 lb Brussels sprouts, halved
- 2 tablespoons olive oil
- Balsamic glaze
- Salt & pepper to taste

**Preparation**:
- Toss Brussels sprouts in olive oil, salt, and pepper.

- Roast until golden, then sprinkle with balsamic glaze.

# 6. Gingered Carrot Soup

*Ingredients*:

- 1 pound carrots, chopped
- 1 onion, chopped
- 2 teaspoons fresh ginger, grated
- Vegetable broth
- Coconut milk
- Salt and pepper to taste

**Preparation**:

1. Sauté carrots, onion, and ginger.
2. Add vegetable broth and cook until veggies are soft.
3. Blend until smooth, then add in coconut milk.

## 7. Baked Apples with Cinnamon

*Ingredients*:

- 4 apples, cored and halved
- 2 tablespoons melted coconut oil
- Cinnamon and nutmeg to taste

**Preparation**:

1. Preheat the oven to 375°F (190°C).
2. Brush apples with warmed coconut oil and sprinkle with cinnamon and nutmeg.
3. Bake until tender.

## Tips for a Reflux-Friendly Feast

**Lean Proteins**: Opt for lean meats like turkey or fish to lower fat content.

**Herbs and Spices**: Flavor foods using herbs and mild spices instead of acidic or spicy ingredients.

**Smaller Portions**: Enjoy smaller, more frequent meals to prevent overeating and lessen strain on the stomach.

**Water with Lemon**: Stay hydrated with water flavored with a touch of lemon instead of acidic drinks.

These dishes give a combination of tastes and textures while reducing frequent causes for acid reflux. Tailor them to your interests and dietary requirements for a joyful and reflux-friendly Christmas event.

# CHAPTER 25: CELEBRATION DESSERTS WITHOUT THE DISCOMFORT

Indulging in tasty treats during celebrations doesn't have to end in agony for individuals struggling with acid reflux. Here are some celebratory dessert choices that are mild on the digestive system:

# 1. Baked Apples with Oat Crumble

*Ingredients*:

- 4 apples, cored and sliced
- 1/2 cup rolled oats
- 1/4 cup almond flour
- 2 tablespoons melted coconut oil
- 1 teaspoon cinnamon
- 1 tablespoon honey (optional)

**Preparation**:

1. Preheat the oven to 375°F (190°C).
2. Place apple slices in a baking tray.
3. In a bowl, combine oats, almond flour, melted coconut oil, and cinnamon.
4. Sprinkle the oat mixture over the apples.
5. Drizzle with honey if desired.
6. Bake until the apples are soft and the crumble is golden.

## 2. Banana and Almond Butter Bites

*Ingredients*:

- 2 bananas, cut
- 2 tablespoons almond butter
- Unsweetened shredded coconut for garnish

**Preparation**:

1. Spread almond butter on banana slices.
2. Sprinkle with shredded coconut.
3. Arrange on a serving plate.

## 3. Chia Seed Pudding with Berries

*Ingredients*:

- 1/4 cup chia seeds
- 1 cup almond milk
- 1 teaspoon vanilla extract
- Mixed berries for topping

**Preparation**:

1. Mix chia seeds, almond milk, and vanilla essence in a dish.
2. Refrigerate for at least 2 hours or until it reaches pudding consistency.
3. Top with mixed berries before serving.

## 4. Pumpkin Pie Smoothie

*Ingredients*:

- 1/2 cup canned pumpkin puree
- 1/2 banana
- 1/2 cup almond milk

- 1/2 teaspoon pumpkin pie spice
- Ice cubes

**Preparation**:

1. Blend all ingredients until smooth.
2. Pour into a glass and sprinkle with extra pumpkin pie spice if desired.

# 5. Coconut and Almond Bliss Balls

*Ingredients*:

- 1 cup shredded coconut
- 1/2 cup almond flour
- 2 tablespoons coconut oil, melted
- 1 tablespoon maple syrup
- 1/2 teaspoon vanilla essence

**Preparation**:

1. Mix shredded coconut, almond flour, melted coconut oil, maple syrup, and vanilla essence in a bowl.
2. Form little balls and chill until hard.

## Tips for Reflux-Friendly Desserts

**Low-Fat Dairy Alternatives**: Use almond or coconut milk instead of standard milk in recipes.

**Moderate Sweeteners**: Opt for natural sweeteners like honey or maple syrup in moderation.

**Avoid Citrus**: Minimize the usage of citrus fruits or seek low-acid kinds.

**Ginger Infusion**: Ginger has anti-inflammatory effects; explore ginger-infused sweets.

**Portion Control**: Enjoy sweets in smaller quantities to minimize overeating.

These celebratory treats give a delicious conclusion without creating acid reflux symptoms. Remember to listen to your body and adjust recipes depending on your individual nutritional requirements and tastes. Celebrate heartily while keeping digestive comfort in mind!

# PART 7

# TIPS FOR LONG-TERM SUCCESS

# CHAPTER 26: MAINTAINING A REFLUX-FRIENDLY LIFESTYLE

Maintaining a reflux-friendly lifestyle goes beyond merely avoiding trigger foods. It is a comprehensive approach that covers food choices, lifestyle behaviors, and mindful practices to nurture digestive health and lessen the effect of acid reflux. Here's a complete guide that contains unique and deep insights backed by up-to-date scientific facts.

## Dietary Considerations

**1. Balanced Nutrition**: Strive for a well-rounded diet that contains a range of fruits, vegetables, lean meats, and complete grains. This not only offers critical nutrients but also aids to general digestive well-being.

A balanced diet promotes optimum gut function and helps avoid overconsumption of particular food categories that may provoke acid reflux.

**2. Mindful Eating**: Adopt mindful eating techniques by enjoying each mouthful, chewing properly, and paying attention to hunger and fullness indicators. This strategy promotes digestion and reduces overeating.

Mindful eating has been related to enhanced digestion and decreased feelings of gastrointestinal discomfort.

# Lifestyle Habits

**3. Regular Physical Activity**: Engage in regular exercise, such as walking, running, or yoga. Exercise enhances general well-being and aids to weight control, lowering the risk of excess abdominal pressure.

Physical exercise has been related with a decreased prevalence of gastroesophageal reflux disease (GERD) and helps improve symptoms in those already afflicted.

**4. Posture Awareness**: Maintain excellent posture, particularly before and after meals, to decrease intra-abdominal pressure. Avoid slouching or laying down shortly after eating. Proper posture helps digestive health by lowering the probability of stomach acid leaking back into the oesophagus.

# Stress Management

**5. Mind-Body Techniques**: Incorporate stress management strategies such as meditation, deep breathing exercises, or progressive muscle relaxation into your regimen. Stress might increase acid reflux symptoms. The gut-brain axis plays a vital role in the link between stress and gastrointestinal health. Mind-body techniques may favorably alter this connection.

**6. Adequate Sleep**: Prioritize adequate and quality sleep. Establish a regular sleep regimen and avoid heavy meals close to bedtime to decrease nocturnal acid reflux. Inadequate sleep has been connected with an increased risk of GERD, stressing the need of prioritizing sufficient sleep for digestive health.

## Hydration and Beverages

**7. Water with Lemon**: Stay hydrated with water, and try adding a touch of lemon. Lemon-infused water may be a delightful, low-acid alternative to acidic drinks. Citrus drinks may add to acid reflux; consequently, drinking water with a touch of lemon delivers hydration without the acidity.

**8. Limiting Trigger Beverages**: Reduce or eliminate caffeinated and carbonated drinks. Opt for herbal teas or non-acidic choices to lessen the danger of acid reflux. Caffeine and carbonation may relax the lower esophageal sphincter, enabling stomach acid to seep back into the oesophagus.

## Sustainable Practices

**9. Constant Pattern**: Establish a constant daily pattern for food, exercise, and sleep. Regularity aids digestive processes and helps avoid disturbances that might lead to acid reflux. Consistency in everyday activities significantly improves digestive health by supporting regularity in digestion and metabolism.

**10. Individualized Approach**: Recognize that each individual may have distinct triggers and reactions to lifestyle circumstances. Keep a diet and symptom record to spot trends and modify your reflux-friendly lifestyle appropriately. Personalized approaches to food and lifestyle adjustments are crucial since causes might vary substantially across people.

Sustaining a reflux-friendly lifestyle means incorporating fresh, science-backed ideas into regular routines. By combining balanced diet, mindful eating, stress management, and smart lifestyle choices, people may create an environment that promotes digestive health and lessens the effect of acid reflux. This holistic and individualized approach provides a complete plan for long-term well-being and comfort. Always speak with healthcare specialists for specific recommendations based on unique health situations.

# CHAPTER 27: TRACKING AND ADJUSTING FOR PERSONALIZED SUCCESS

Creating a specific and effective strategy to controlling acid reflux entails a constant process of recording, assessing, and modifying numerous lifestyle variables. By adopting a personalized approach based on individual reactions, people may attain more control over their symptoms. This creative and informative handbook includes up-to-date scientific knowledge to help people on their quest toward tailored success in acid reflux treatment.

**1. Symptom Tracking**: To commence on a tailored strategy, start by closely recording acid reflux symptoms and their likely sources. Maintain a comprehensive journal noting meals, drinks, stress levels, sleep patterns, and other pertinent activities.

Techniques such as mobile applications or digital journals may permit real-time monitoring, providing a more precise examination of patterns and relationships. Studies show that maintaining a symptom diary is a good way for identifying specific triggers, leading to individualized acid reflux care regimens.

**2. Identifying Triggers**: Once a sizable dataset is acquired, evaluate the recorded information to detect repeating trends. Look for links between certain meals, activities, or stress levels and the beginning or severity of acid reflux symptoms. This tailored understanding creates the basis for targeted modifications.

Recent study underlines the heterogeneity of triggers across people, stressing the significance of individualized diagnosis to better symptom treatment.

**3. Customizing Dietary Choices**: Utilize the data acquired to adjust nutritional choices depending on individual triggers. This may entail removing or decreasing particular foods known to increase acid reflux symptoms. Experiment with alternate ingredients and cooking techniques, introducing innovative, reflux-friendly foods into your routine.

**4. Optimizing Meal Time**: Adjust meal time depending on recorded trends. Consider dividing meals into smaller, more regular servings throughout the day to minimize overeating. Additionally, avoid heavy meals close to sleep, minimizing the chance of nocturnal acid reflux.

Studies demonstrate that changing meal time and quantity control significantly affect symptoms, underlining the relevance of temporal considerations in acid reflux therapy.

**5. Mind-Body Approaches for Stress Management**: Evaluate stress levels reported in the tracking process and use individualized stress management approaches. Incorporate mindfulness meditation, deep breathing techniques, or progressive muscle relaxation depending on individual preferences and efficacy. Emerging evidence supports the significance of mind-body approaches in lowering stress-related symptoms, particularly those connected with acid reflux.

**6. Regular Exercise Tailored to Individual Preferences**: Examine the influence of exercise on acid reflux symptoms by analyzing monitored data. Customize a workout plan based on personal preferences and tolerances, integrating activities that offer pleasure and relaxation while contributing to general well-being. Personalized exercise programs have shown benefit in controlling acid reflux symptoms, underlining the necessity for personalized physical activity.

**7. Sleep Hygiene Adjustments**: Review sleep patterns established in the monitoring process and make modifications for individual success. Ensure appropriate sleep time and try elevating the upper body during sleep to lessen the risk of nocturnal acid reflux. Studies show the association between poor sleep and increased acid reflux symptoms, stressing the necessity of individualized sleep hygiene changes.

**8. Consistent Monitoring and Reassessment:** Implement a constant monitoring and reassessment process. Regularly review the monitoring procedure to assess the success of tailored modifications. Be flexible to adjusting methods depending on developing lifestyle circumstances and individual reactions. Longitudinal monitoring and evaluation are crucial to sustaining good acid reflux therapy, harmonizing with the dynamic character of individual responses.

Measuring and modifying for individualized success in acid reflux therapy entails a rigorous and changing procedure. By employing up-to-date scientific knowledge, people may walk a route personalized to their particular triggers and reactions. This novel technique not only promotes symptom management but also encourages people to actively engage in their health and well-being. Always consult with healthcare specialists for individualized advice and help in the treatment of acid reflux.

# BONUSES

## THE 28 DAY MEAL PLANS

Creating a 28-day meal plan for acid reflux requires choosing meals that are mild on the digestive system and limiting triggers that might increase symptoms. Here's a full 28-day meal plan with recipes and nutritional facts to help control acid reflux:

## Week 1

*Day 1:* Breakfast hash with eggs, potatoes, broccoli, spinach, and mushrooms; Veggie sandwich on whole wheat bread with hummus, cucumber, greens, and red onions; Baked ginger salmon served with roasted broccoli and brown rice

***Day 2:*** Rice Chex cereal with sliced banana and almond milk; Tuna salad wrap; Gluten-free chicken spaghetti

***Day 3:*** Green smoothie prepared with coconut milk, spinach, mango, and banana; Peanut butter and honey sandwich with baked potato chips; Baked chicken thighs over rice

***Day 4:*** Simple rice pudding prepared with cooked rice, rice milk, and sugar; Boiled eggs with crackers and applesauce; Turkey meatballs over gluten-free spaghetti

***Day 5:*** Peanut butter smoothie prepared with milk, yogurt, peanut butter, and banana; Meatball sub; Ginger rice, sautéed mushrooms & carrots, and grilled chicken breast or turkey

***Day 6:*** Whole grain toast with almond butter and sliced pear; Quinoa salad with mixed veggies and grilled chicken; Baked salmon with steamed asparagus and quinoa

***Day 7:*** Oatmeal with sliced banana and berries; Grilled veggie and hummus sandwich; Turkey and vegetable soup

## Week 2

***Day 8:*** Greek yogurt with honey and fruit; Quinoa and veggie salad; Lemon herb grilled chicken with roasted sweet potatoes

***Day 9:*** Scrambled eggs with spinach and feta cheese; Turkey and avocado wrap; Baked cod with quinoa and steamed asparagus

Day 10: Chia seed pudding with chopped strawberries; Chicken Caesar salad; Turkey and vegetable soup

*Day 11:* Whole grain toast with almond butter and sliced pear; Greek salad with grilled chicken; Baked salmon with quinoa and steamed broccoli

*Day 12:* Blueberry banana smoothie; Veggie wrap with hummus; Grilled chicken with roasted veggies

*Day 13:* Mango lovely cream; Tuna salad on whole grain toast; Turkey meatballs with whole grain noodles

*Day 14:* Banana oat pancakes; Quinoa and black bean salad; Lemon herb grilled chicken with roasted sweet potatoes

## Week 3

*Day 15:* Overnight oats with mixed berries; Greek yogurt with honey and nuts; Baked chicken with quinoa and steamed asparagus

*Day 16:* Avocado toast with whole grain bread; Turkey and veggie wrap; Baked salmon with quinoa and roasted veggies

*Day 17*: Green smoothie with spinach, pineapple, and banana; Quinoa salad with mixed veggies and grilled chicken; Lemon herb grilled chicken with roasted sweet potatoes

*Day 18*: Chia seed pudding with sliced strawberries; Greek salad with grilled chicken; Turkey meatballs with whole grain noodles

*Day 19*: Whole grain toast with almond butter and sliced pear; Veggie wrap with hummus; Baked cod with quinoa and steamed asparagus

*Day 20:* Blueberry banana smoothie; Tuna salad on whole grain toast; Grilled chicken with roasted veggies

*Day 21*: Banana oat pancakes; Quinoa and black bean salad; Baked salmon with quinoa and steamed broccoli

## Week 4

*Day 22*: Overnight oats with mixed berries; Greek yogurt with honey and nuts; Baked chicken with quinoa and steamed asparagus

***Day 23***: Avocado toast with whole grain bread; Turkey and veggie wrap; Lemon herb grilled chicken with roasted sweet potatoes

***Day 24***: Green smoothie with spinach, pineapple, and banana; Quinoa salad with mixed veggies and grilled chicken; Baked salmon with quinoa and roasted veggies

***Day 25***: Chia seed pudding with chopped strawberries; Greek salad with grilled chicken; Turkey meatballs with whole grain noodles

***Day 26***: Whole grain toast with almond butter and sliced pear; Veggie wrap with hummus; Baked cod with quinoa and steamed asparagus

***Day 27***: Blueberry banana smoothie; Tuna salad on whole grain toast; Grilled chicken with roasted veggies

***Day 28***: Banana oat pancakes; Quinoa and black bean salad; Lemon herb grilled chicken with roasted sweet potatoes

This 28-day meal plan contains a range of nutrient-dense meals while avoiding known culprits for acid reflux. It's crucial to change portion quantities and components depending on your individual tolerance and preferences. Always talk with a healthcare practitioner or a trained nutritionist before making substantial changes to your diet.

# GROCERY SHOPPING TIPS

Grocery shopping for acid reflux-friendly meals may be a major aspect of controlling symptoms. Here are some ideas to help you navigate the grocery shop and make smart choices:

**Focus on Fresh Produce**: Opt for a range of fresh fruits and vegetables. Bananas, pears, potatoes, broccoli, cabbage, carrots, celery, and leafy greens like spinach and kale are typically prescribed for those with acid reflux. These components are versatile and may be utilized in a broad variety of cuisines.

**Whole Grains**: Look for whole grain alternatives such as whole grain pasta, whole grain crackers, and brown rice. These deliver fiber and nutrition while being mild on the digestive tract.

**Lean Proteins**: Choose lean cuts of meat, poultry, and fish. Incorporating protein sources like chicken, turkey, and fish may help balance meals and supply critical nutrients.

**Dairy substitutes**: For individuals sensitive to dairy, try dairy substitutes such as almond milk or oat milk. These may be used in smoothies, cereals, or eaten on their own.

**Healthy Fats**: Include sources of healthy fats such as olive oil, almonds, and seeds. These may be used in cooking, baking, or as toppings for salads and yogurt.

**Portion Control**: When food shopping, examine the size of the things you are purchasing. Opt for fewer servings of things that may provoke acid reflux symptoms.

**Read Labels**: Be wary of extra sugars, artificial additives, and preservatives in packaged goods. Choose things with minimum chemicals and substances that you can identify.

**Keep a Food Diary**: Consider keeping a food diary to document how your body responds to various meals. Note down what you consume, the time of day, and any symptoms you have. This might help you identify trigger foods and make educated decisions.

**Seek Professional Advice**: Always talk with a healthcare practitioner or a trained nutritionist before making substantial changes to your diet. They may make unique advice based on your individual demands and health situation.

**Experiment and Adjust**: Everyone's body reacts differently to meals. It's vital to experiment with various meals and notice how your body responds. Over time, you may change your shopping list depending on your specific experiences.

By implementing these guidelines into your grocery shopping routine, you may make educated decisions and pick foods that are soft on the digestive system, possibly minimizing the frequency and intensity of acid reflux symptoms.

# CONCLUSION

In the path toward efficient acid reflux treatment, the "Acid Reflux Diet Cookbook for Beginners" serves as a thorough guide, delivering not just recipes but a specific roadmap for sustainable relief. As we close this informative book, remember that controlling acid reflux is not a one-size-fits-all approach. The strength is in the details—the rigorous monitoring, intelligent modifications, and the individualized plans.

This cookbook goes beyond the usual, presenting a creative and precise method that encourages people to retake control over their digestive health. From grasping the complexities of trigger detection to the skill of making reflux-friendly foods, every page is a step toward a life free from the misery of acid reflux.

As you begin on this transforming journey, I ask you to share your experiences and observations. Your input is not simply a review but a light for those seeking healing. Let your voice enhance the worth of this book so that more folks can discover the depth of information inside its pages. Together, let's establish a community of empowered people actively designing their path toward digestive well-being.

Thank you for being part of this adventure. Your review is not just a gesture; it's a contribution to a collaborative effort to promote awareness and help individuals navigate the problems of acid reflux.

*Happy reading, exploring, and loving the road to a reflux-free life!*

# About the Author

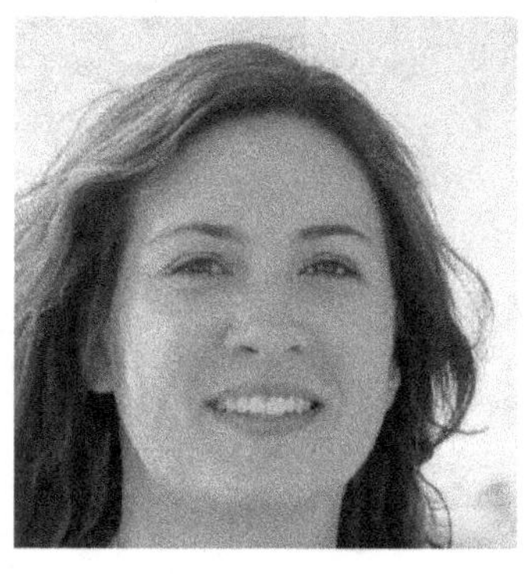 Dr. Dorothy S. Richard is a passionate and devoted advocate for holistic well-being. With a foundation in medicine and a diploma in nutrition, she has spent her career helping people find the keys to a better, happier life. Her path into the realm of health and nutrition was prompted by a highly personal experience—her aunt's struggle with cancer in 1983. This important event kindled Dorothy's lifetime passion to studying the possibility of holistic approaches to health.

Raised in the stunning vistas of Alaska, Dorothy learnt the significance of simple, natural choices in promoting healthy living. Her personal challenges with health difficulties, including genetic predispositions and less-than-ideal eating habits, spurred her resolve to harness the power of right nutrition and mindful eating.

Dorothy is not simply a doctor; she is a friend, a mentor, and a light of hope for individuals wanting to live their best lives. Beyond her professional successes, she spends her life with Steven Richard, a retired psychologist, and their three cherished children. Together, they have developed a life based on holistic wellbeing and happiness.

Through her profession and her writing, she tries to make the route to health an easy and joyous trip for everyone.

www.ingramcontent.com/pod-product-compliance
Lightning Source LLC
Chambersburg PA
CBHW070923260726
48661CB00003B/804